The Lean Machine

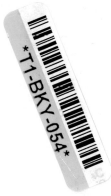

The Lean Machine

David Luna's Guide to Total Fitness and the Sensible Diet

By David Luna

Photographs by Patrick Nagatani

PEACE PRESS

Peace Press, Inc.
3828 Willat Avenue
Culver City, California 90230

9 8 7 6 5 4 3 2 1

Cover photograph by Patrick Nagatani.
Typesetting by Freedmen's Organization, Los Angeles.
Printed in the United States of America by Peace Press.

Library of Congress Cataloging in Publication Data

Luna, David, 1947–
   The lean machine.

   Bibliography: p.
   Includes index.
   1. Physical fitness.   2. Exercise.
3. Diet.   4. Nutrition.   I. Title.
RA781.L88   613.7   79-89792
ISBN 0-915238-34-9 (paper)
ISBN 0-915238-36-5 (cloth)

To my family, Ida Jaqua, and my students. . . . .

We squander health
In search of wealth;
We scheme and toil and save;
Then squander wealth
In search of health
And all we get's a grave.
We live and boast of what we own;
We die and only get a stone.
    Anonymous

Contents

Acknowledgements

I want to say thank you to a lot of beautiful people who worked with me on this book—people who contributed their time, energy, ideas, and expertise.

First, thanks to Ida Jaqua, nutrition professor at Los Angeles Valley College, for giving me the groundwork and fundamentals in nutrition and dietetics, and also for assisting with the manuscript. Her time and energy proved to be invaluable.

Secondly, I'd like to express my thanks to the entire staff at Peace Press. Special thanks to Dinah Portner who spent many hours editing this book—she made working on this project a delight. Thanks also to Deborah Lott for her editorial assistance; Bonnie Mettler for art direction and design; and Bob Zaugh, Janis Zaccaria, Melinda Grubbauer, George Fuller, and everyone who participated in the production of this book for their individual contributions.

Thanks to Dr. George Elmstrom of the American Optometric Association and International Academy of Preventive Medicine, who provided an endless source of ideas and information. I would also like to thank one of the top cardiologists in the country, Dr. Harold Bailey, Fellow of the American College of Surgeons, who cordially allowed me to absorb a river of information every time we met.

A special note of thanks to Stephanie Floyd, the lady who served as the catalyst for the writing of this project.

I'd also like to acknowledge and thank a good friend who served as an advisor, Dr. James Gernert, member of the American Board of Urology and a Fellow of the American College of Surgeons.

The list of special people would not be complete without a special thank you to Adrian Thornberry, President of the International Health Club, one of the finest health facilities in Los Angeles, for providing me with a training ground which allowed me to be innovative. I'd also like to thank Roz Kirby Sullivan, of the Beverly Hills Health Club, for her faith and confidence in me, and for giving me my start in this business many years ago; and, of course, Jim Heflin, fitness and nutritional consultant, for getting me started on the right foot.

I'd also like to express my appreciation to Patrick Nagatani for the excellent photography and to Deborah Bledsoe for assisting with the rope jumping photographs. Additional photography was provided by Erik Stern and Gordon Layne. Thanks also to Scott Smith, editor of *Vegetarian Times* and health food industry consultant; and to Robert Yudelson, D.D.S., for the research studies he provided relating to refined carbohydrates and tooth decay.

Special thanks to Casey Kaysen whose frankness, depth, and new dimensions have been a step to higher consciousness and awareness in *all* aspects of life.

Thanks also to Marlene Brause for all her encouragement and assistance.

Then there are my students. All I can say is . . . you have taught me well. Stay ''positively addicted'' and remember what I've always told you:

THE ONLY RESTRICTIONS AND LIMITATIONS IN LIFE ARE THOSE WHICH WE CREATE FOR OURSELVES.

DAVID LUNA

Introduction

We live in a society that is gradually self-destructing. This is an age when much of the food that we eat is nutritionally deficient, the air that we breathe is polluted, the water that we drink is impure, and the lifestyle that we lead is becoming more and more sedentary. With so many obstacles to good health facing us at every turn, it is easy to see why so many people throw up their hands at the seemingly hopeless task of living more healthful lives.

Does it come as any surprise to discover that 30% of the American population is obese? That's one out of every three people! Cigarette smoking is another example. Has the label warning that tobacco may be hazardous to one's health deterred smokers? The average smoker in this country smokes approximately 4,000 cigarettes annually.

Our stressful, sedentary urban lives are not particularly helpful either. According to Dr. Laurence Morehouse, head of the Human Performance Laboratory at UCLA, it has been calculated that a person who is inactive for three days will lose 5% of his or her strength and a person who does not exercise for one month will lose 80%. The average male is now considered middle-aged by the time he reaches the age of twenty-seven. One of the reasons for this is that most people live as foreigners in their own bodies. They don't understand, pay attention to or listen to their bodies. Even when the warning signals strike, there is a tendency to disregard them.

Why all the self-abuse? Why the neglect? Part of the problem stems from our inability to accept the fact that how we live has a direct relationship to when and how we die. We all live with a false sense of security. We always assume it's going to happen to the "other guy." The "other guy" is going to get a coronary or have an accident, but not us. This denial is both unrealistic and dangerous. Fortunately, good health is not as impossible to maintain as it may seem. Only if we remain conscious that harm can come to us, can we begin to effect change. By taking a more realistic approach, we can make the changes that are necessary to reduce the risks to our health and increase our general well-being.

Just as negative emotions produce negative chemical changes in the body, positive emotions are connected to positive chemical changes. Happiness is a habit, just as unhappiness is a habit. It's easy to blame unhappiness on external causes, when in reality we create our own mental and emotional states simply by what we choose to do or not do. If we can make ourselves miserable, we can also make ourselves happier and healthier— and without a tremendous amount of effort.

It never ceases to amaze me how some people take better care of their automobiles than they do of their bodies. They make sure that the car is well tuned, that the oil is changed, that it is lubricated, and that they use the best type of fuel. The irony of all this is that they then turn around and run themselves down, stuff themselves with junk foods all day, abuse themselves with drugs or alcohol at night, and then try to compensate the following morning by having a "well-balanced" breakfast which will probably consist of black coffee, sweet rolls, a few cigarettes, and maybe even a few "uppers" to get themselves going. In the meantime, the car is running smoothly. It had a good night's rest in the garage. It didn't wake up feeling nauseated and sick, or with a congested carburetor. If anything, it feels like it's ready for another ten thousand miles—and, with certain important adjustments, so can you.

The Lean Machine is a program for fitness and nutrition that can be easily incorporated into your daily routine, no matter how busy you may be. The guide to stretching, rope jumping, nutrition and cardiovascular fitness that you hold in your hands will provide you with the most up-to-date information available for getting into shape and staying there. The rest is up to you.

1. STRETCHING

Stretching is an integral part of all the fitness and training programs that I teach. Its purpose is to reduce injuries and to increase flexibility. Stretching should be practiced before *all* strenuous exercise and in some cases afterwards as well. Pre-exercise stretching is the most important. If you are especially tight or engage in muscle-building activities, five minutes of post-exercise stretching is also recommended.

Stretching is both natural and automatic. We often stretch unconsciously upon waking or after sitting for an extended period of time. If anything, it's unnatural *not* to stretch. One of the most important benefits of stretching is learning to relax—an excellent remedy to the daily stresses to which most of us are subject.

Above all, stretching should be fun and comfortable. It should not be painful. If it becomes painful, then you are automatically defeating your purpose by causing the muscles to tense and tighten. This creates a reactive contraction of the muscle tissue.

You can stretch any time and anywhere: talking on the telephone, taking a bath, working at a desk, watching television, before and after participating in a sports activity, before and after rest or sleep, while reading a book.

Who Should Stretch

Workers, players, young people, old people, men, women, boys and girls—everyone should stretch. This is recommended not only for training purposes, but for the reduction of injuries, particularly those of the lower back and hamstrings. A study conducted by Dr. Sawny Gaston at Columbia Presbyterian Hospital in New York found that over 83% of the 3,000 apparently healthy subjects they tested, failed one or more measures of minimum strength and flexibility of the key postural muscles.[1] The results of this study give us an indication of how poorly most urban Americans fare in the area of strength and flexibility.

This is one reason why it's so important to stretch on a regular basis. If the muscles in the lower back, for example, are weak or tight from tension, then it will be necessary to stretch and build up surrounding muscles such as the hamstrings, the buttocks, and the lower abdominals to help bear the load and prevent structural imbalances. This can only be done gradually over a long period of time.

It is important to note that *everyone* is capable of stretching, men and women alike. All we need to do is to observe male gymnasts, dancers or yoga practitioners—not to mention most

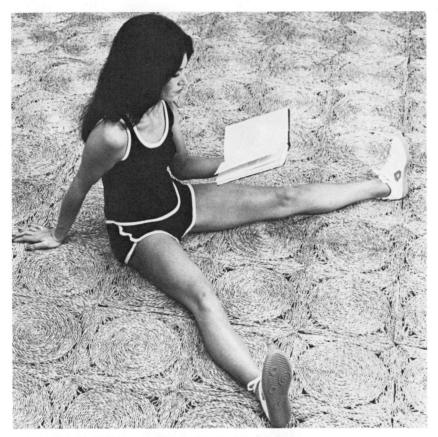

To stretch adductors and hamstrings while reading or watching television, sit with legs apart, toes pointed toward ceiling.

Stretching Exercises for Running, Jogging and General Toning

I stretch every day and never start my workouts without doing a minimum of five to ten minutes of stretching. Three to four times a week, I go through all of the stretching exercises which are illustrated in this chapter. The complete routine takes about forty minutes.

I cannot emphasize enough the importance of regular stretching. Stretching is a required activity for all my students. It doesn't matter whether they are lawyers, truck drivers, physicians, world class or professional athletes—they all must stretch.

One year, I was working with Eddie Bell of the New York Jets. He had just been traded to the Green Bay Packers and came to see me that summer for a conditioning program. I put him on a weight-training regimen that also included rope jumping, jogging and stretching. He followed it regularly, with the exception of the stretching. When it came time for him to leave for camp, I wished him well, still unaware that he had not done any stretching. He had gotten himself into excellent condition, but he was as tight as a knot. As you might have predicted, when he got to camp and started training, he pulled one muscle after another. Three weeks later, he was back in Los Angeles and out of a job.

So, whether you are a professional athlete or not, if you stretch regularly before participating in any physical activity, you will be much more likely to minimize your chances of injury.

Stretching should involve both agonistic and antagonistic muscles. The agonistic muscles initiate movement while the antagonistic muscles inhibit movement. There is a tendency, particularly among runners, to develop strong calf muscles, but to have rather weak anterior tibial muscles (shin muscles). This is one of the primary causes of *shin splints* (inflammation of the

fine athletes—to realize that men can be tremendously flexible. Yet men in our culture have traditionally placed more emphasis on muscle building, which has a tendency to shorten the muscles, thus increasing the need for stretching even more. We are all capable of an amazingly wide range of strength and elasticity. Most of us never even get close to our full potential for either.

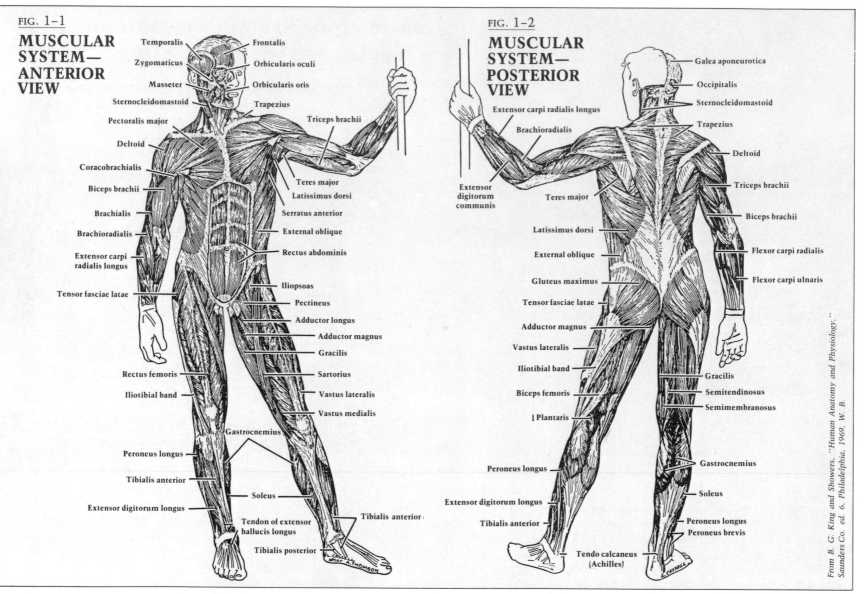

MUSCULAR SYSTEM— ANTERIOR VIEW

Temporalis
Zygomaticus
Masseter
Sternocleidomastoid
Pectoralis major
Deltoid
Coracobrachialis
Biceps brachii
Brachialis
Brachioradialis
Extensor carpi radialis longus
Tensor fasciae latae
Rectus femoris
Iliotibial band
Gastrocnemius
Peroneus longus
Tibialis anterior
Extensor digitorum longus
Tendon of extensor hallucis longus
Tibialis posterior

Frontalis
Orbicularis oculi
Orbicularis oris
Trapezius
Triceps brachii
Teres major
Latissimus dorsi
Serratus anterior
External oblique
Rectus abdominis
Iliopsoas
Pectineus
Adductor longus
Adductor magnus
Gracilis
Sartorius
Vastus lateralis
Vastus medialis
Soleus
Tibialis anterior

FIG. 1-2

MUSCULAR SYSTEM— POSTERIOR VIEW

Extensor carpi radialis longus
Brachioradialis
Extensor digitorum communis
Teres major
Latissimus dorsi
External oblique
Gluteus maximus
Tensor fasciae latae
Adductor magnus
Vastus lateralis
Iliotibial band
Biceps femoris
Plantaris
Peroneus longus
Extensor digitorum longus
Tibialis anterior

Galea aponeurotica
Occipitalis
Sternocleidomastoid
Trapezius
Deltoid
Triceps brachii
Biceps brachii
Flexor carpi radialis
Flexor carpi ulnaris
Gracilis
Semitendinosus
Semimembranosus
Gastrocnemius
Soleus
Peroneus longus
Peroneus brevis
Tendo calcaneus (Achilles)

From B. G. King and Showers, "Human Anatomy and Physiology." Saunders Co. ed. 6, Philadelphia. 1969. W. B.

4

muscles surrounding the shin area). The exercises presented here are designed to stretch both muscle groups, to aid in the prevention of these problems for more efficient and safer rope jumping and running, as well as for general toning. These stretches concentrate primarily on three areas: (1) achilles tendons, calves and insteps; (2) hamstrings (back of thighs) and quadriceps (front of thighs); and (3) the lower back.

My own personal stretching routine consists of the entire set of twenty stretches illustrated in this chapter. If you have not been exercising regularly, you may want to start by only practicing the first ten exercises for two or three weeks, then gradually begin to add one new stretch each week until you incorporate them all. If you have a time limit and cannot do the entire routine, it is better to do only part rather than none at all. In any case, do not reduce the length of time that each position is held. Hold each one, to whatever degree is most comfortable, for thirty seconds, or count to ten very slowly. If you cannot hold the position for thirty seconds, then you are probably doing a ''drastic stretch,'' i.e., overstretching beyond your limits. Ease into a position you can maintain for that length of time and allow yourself to progress forward slowly with each practice session.

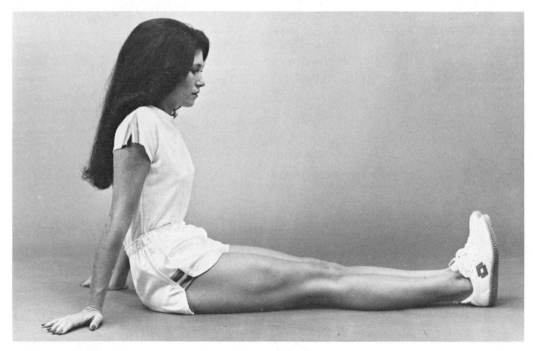

Keep feet dorsiflexed (bent upward at ankles), as shown, during stretching exercises, unless indicated otherwise.

The following pointers will help you to improve your stretching program and to progress at a much faster rate:

Do's and Don'ts for Stretching

DO keep in mind that stretching is a way to relax and to become more in tune with your body.

DO maintain slow and rhythmic breathing in order to stretch more effectively.

DO keep feet dorsiflexed (see illustration), unless otherwise indicated, to get the maximum benefit from each stretch.

DO hold each stretch for thirty seconds or count to ten very slowly.

DO ease into the stretch. If you feel pain, you have gone too far—back off, relax and enjoy the stretch.

DO move gently and gracefully from one stretch to the next. Avoid abrupt or jerking movements.

DO work towards the goal given with each stretch. Visualize your goal, even if you cannot yet attain it.

DO be patient with yourself. Continuous practice will allow you to come closer and closer to your goals, but some may take years to accomplish.

DON'T hold your breath during any stretch or any other exercise that you may do. Holding your breath may produce an immediate rise in blood pressure, particularly with weight-bearing exercises.

DON'T rush. Stretching is a slow, relaxing, rhythmic process which should not be associated with pressure, tension, or anxiety.

DON'T bounce. Bouncing produces small muscle tears and causes the muscles to contract, which is exactly the opposite of what you are trying to do.

DON'T expect too much too soon. Be alert to the difference between the pull of a comfortable stretch and the pain that can result when you have pulled too far too fast.

DON'T make comparisons with others or try to compete with anyone else while stretching. This is not a contest.

DON'T place emphasis on flexibility in the beginning, but rather on how the stretch *feels*. Stressing flexibility initially may lead to overstretching. Let your body lead you slowly and naturally to its full potential for flexibility.

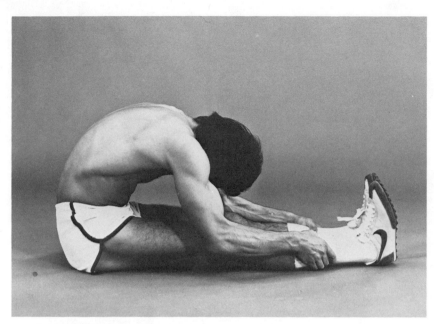

Beginning Back Stretch

The Stretching Routine

The twenty exercises in this routine flow from one to the next in a natural sequence. Start by jogging in place for about a minute, then sit on the floor with your feet extended in front of you. Shake out your legs for about fifteen seconds in this seated position to increase circulation before you begin to stretch.

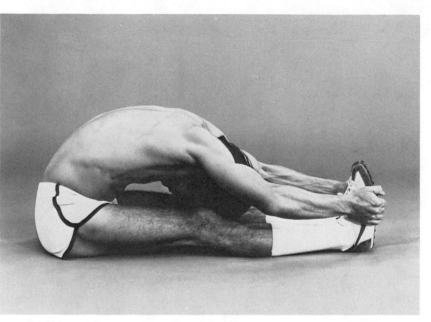

Advanced Back Stretch

1. Back Stretch *(Beginning and Advanced)*

This stretch is for the back of the thighs (hamstrings) and lower back. In this and all of the following exercises: *Move Slowly. Do Not Bounce. Do Not Hold Your Breath. Breathe Normally.*

Sit with feet together, legs extended in front of you.

Slowly, bend forward, holding legs at calves, ankles or feet.

Gently, pull forehead toward knees.

Hold for 30 seconds.

GOAL: To touch forehead to knees, hands grasping feet.

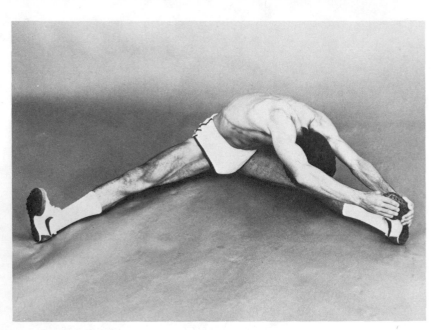

Alternate Leg Pull

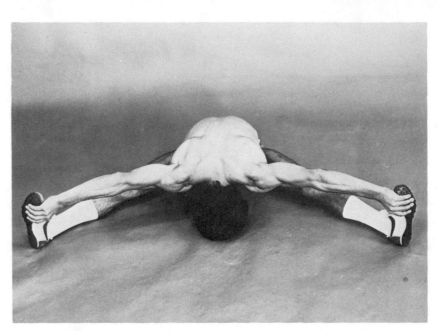

Diamond Stretch

2. Alternate Leg Pull

This stretch is for the back of the thighs (hamstrings) and inner thighs (adductors).

Open legs as wide as possible into a "V" position.

Keep feet dorsiflexed, toes pointing upwards, not out.

Keeping legs straight, reach with both hands toward left foot.

Grasp knee, calf, ankle or foot with both hands.

Hold for 30 seconds.

Repeat on right side.

GOAL: To touch forehead to knee while keeping both legs straight and holding foot with both hands.

3. Diamond Stretch

This stretch is for the back of the thighs (hamstrings), inner thighs (adductors), and lower back.

Sit with back straight, legs apart.

Reach forward to grasp both knees, calves, ankles or feet at once.

Allow head to fall forward toward the floor.

Hold in your most extended position for 30 seconds.

GOAL: To touch top of head to floor, keeping both legs straight, holding feet. *Keep in mind that with daily practice it may take six months to a year to reach your goal.*

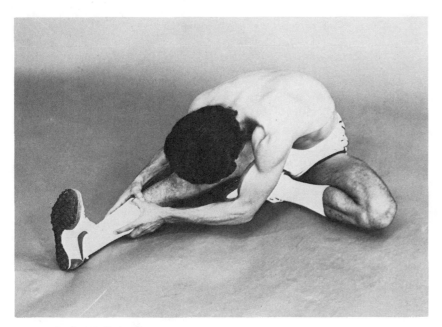

Beginning Half Hurdler

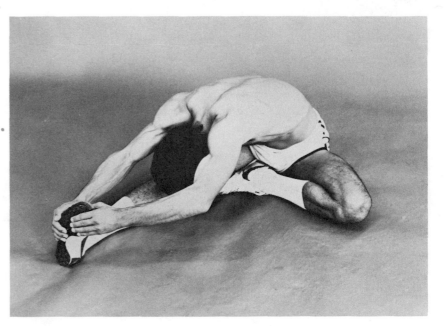

Advanced Half Hurdler

4. Half Hurdler *(Beginning and Advanced)*

This stretch is for the inner thighs (adductors) and for the back of the thighs (hamstrings).

Sit with back straight, keeping legs apart as in previous exercise.

Bend left leg and place sole of foot firmly against right thigh, as shown.

Reach forward and grasp right knee, calf, ankle or foot with both hands, forehead down.

Keep bent knee on floor, or as close to floor as possible.

Hold for 30 seconds.

Move to opposite side slowly and gently, first by straightening left leg out, then bending right knee, and repeat.

GOAL: To touch forehead to knee, keeping extended leg straight, bent knee on floor, and holding foot with both hands.

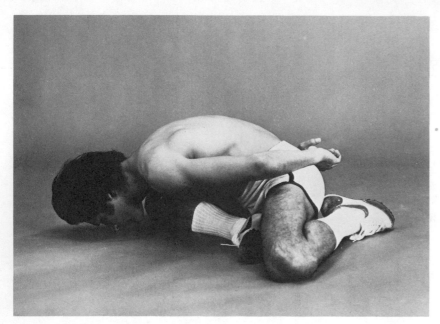

Pinwheel

5. Pinwheel

This stretch is for the back of the thighs (hamstrings), frontal thighs (quadriceps), and lower back.

Remaining in the half hurdler position, sit up straight, keeping right leg bent into left thigh.

Bend left leg behind you, as shown.

Clasp hands behind back, and bend forward, aiming forehead towards floor.

Hold for 30 seconds without bouncing.

Slowly and gently, change sides and repeat.

GOAL: To touch forehead to floor with knees down and hands clasped.

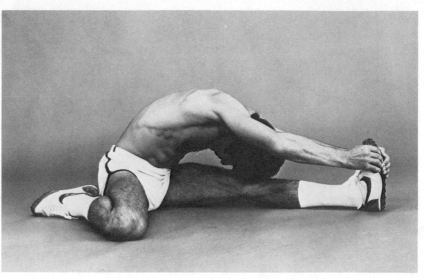

Hurdler

6. Hurdler

This stretch is for the front of the thighs (quadriceps), back of the thighs (hamstrings), and the lower back.

From Pinwheel position, sit up straight.

Keeping right leg bent behind, slowly extend left leg forward, as shown.

Reach forward with both hands to grasp knee, calf, ankle or foot.

Bring forehead as close as possible to extended leg.

Hold for 30 seconds.

Slowly and gently, straighten knee, change sides, and repeat with other leg.

GOAL: To touch forehead to knee, keeping hips and legs on the floor, holding foot with both hands.

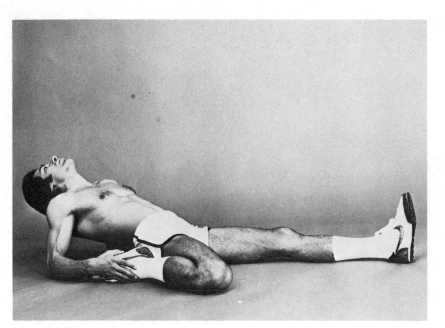

Lay-Back

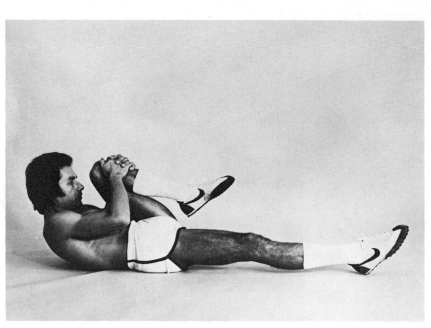

Hip Flexor Stretch

7. Lay-Back

CAUTION: *If you have a back problem, omit this stretch.*

This exercise is for the front of the thighs (quadriceps).

From Hurdler position, release hold on foot and gently lean back as far as possible, resting weight on elbows and forearms in back, as shown.

Make sure that bent knee remains on the floor.

Hold for 30 seconds.

Slowly and gently, lift torso, change sides and repeat with opposite leg.

GOAL: To bring your head and torso all the way to the floor while keeping the bent knee on the floor and extended leg straight.

8. Hip Flexor Stretch

This stretch is for the back of the thighs (hamstrings).

Lie flat on your back with legs extended, feet together.

Raise left knee to the chest.

Grasp knee with both hands and lift head, as shown.

Bring forehead as close to the knee as possible.

Hold for 30 seconds.

Relax, change sides and repeat.

GOAL: To touch forehead to knee while keeping extended leg on the floor.

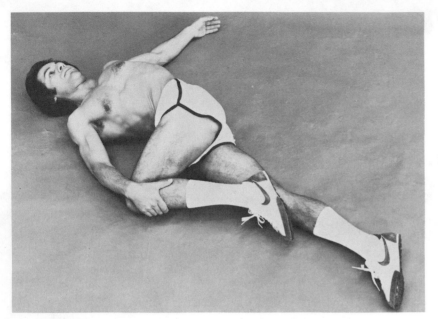

Knee-Over

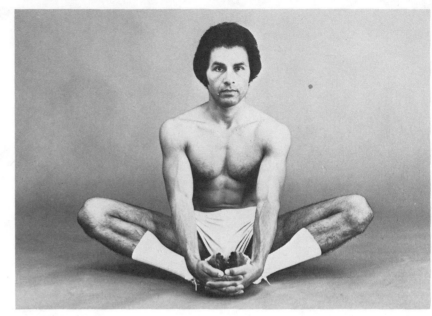

Beginning Butterfly

9. Knee-Over

This stretch is for the lower back and buttocks.

Begin as in previous exercise, lying flat on your back with legs extended.

Lift left knee to chest.

Place right hand on outside of left knee and pull it across body.

Bring bent knee as close to floor as possible.

Keep both shoulders flat on the floor, right leg extended.

Hold for 30 seconds without bouncing.

Return to center and repeat on other side.

GOAL: To touch knee to floor while keeping shoulders flat.

10. Butterfly *(Beginning and Advanced)*

This stretch is for the inner thighs (adductors).

Sit with knees turned out, feet together, back as straight as possible.

Holding feet together with both hands, expand the chest upward and lower the knees as close to the floor as possible.

Hold for 30 seconds.

GOAL: To touch knees to floor.

Advanced position is for inner thighs (adductors) and lower back. Allow head to fall forward slowly towards feet.

GOAL: To touch head to toes and knees to floor.

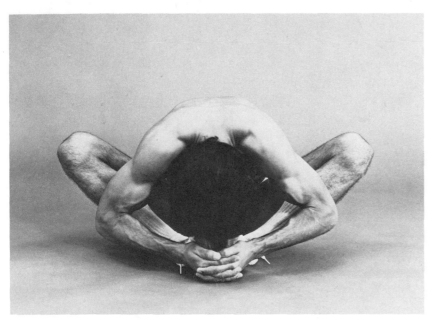

Advanced Butterfly

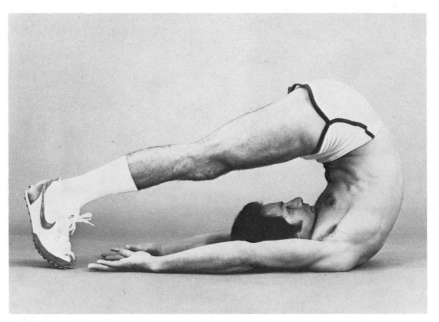

The Plough

11. The Plough

This stretch is for the upper and lower back.

Lie on your back, hands at your sides, palms braced against floor.

Swing your legs up and over your head, gradually lowering them behind your head as shown. Move as slowly as possible.

Pull your arms up over head, reaching toward toes.

Chin is pressed against chest, toes on floor, legs straight as possible.

Do not hold your breath. If you have difficulty breathing while in fully extended position, slowly ease up on stretch by lifting both legs.

Hold for 30 seconds.

GOAL: To touch toes to floor keeping both legs straight.

Come out of the position exactly as instructed (it is important to maintain smoothness and balance): Bend knees and lower them toward head. Return arms to original position, palms down at your sides. Roll forward, arching neck to keep head on floor. Keep the knees bent to prevent lower back injury as you slowly lower both legs to the floor.

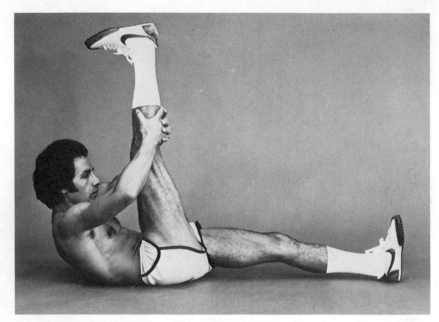

Right Angle Stretch

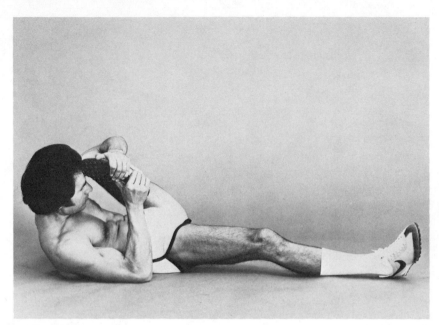

Foot to Forehead

12. Right Angle Stretch

This stretch is for the back of the thighs (hamstrings).

Lie on your back, hands at sides, feet together.

Keeping both legs straight, raise left leg up, aiming bottom of foot to ceiling.

With both hands, grasp raised leg at thigh, moving hands up to calf as you bring head up to meet leg, as shown.

Hold for 30 seconds without bouncing.

Slowly release, return to supine position and repeat with right leg.

GOAL: To touch forehead to knee, keeping both legs straight and lowered leg flat on the floor.

13. Foot to Forehead

This stretch is for the back of the thighs (hamstrings) and the buttocks (gluteal muscles).

From raised leg position of Right Angle Stretch, bend knee of raised leg.

Grasp foot with both hands and bring foot as close to forehead as possible.

Hold for 30 seconds.

Straighten and lower leg slowly. Repeat on opposite side.

GOAL: To touch foot to forehead.

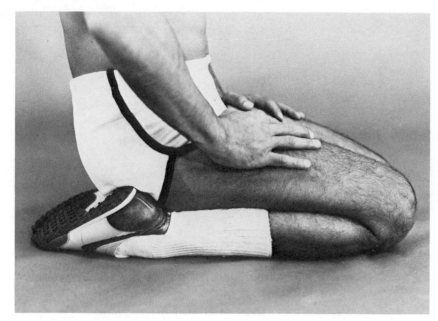

Shin Stretch

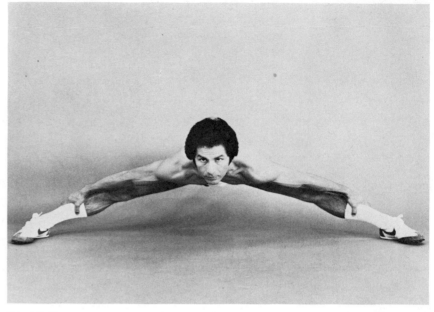

Front Split

14. Shin Stretch

This stretch is for the shins (anterior tibial muscles). It's excellent for helping to prevent shin splints.

Kneel with knees slightly apart, feet behind you.

Top of feet should rest flat on the floor (*not* dorsiflexed for this stretch).

Slowly lower your body to sit on heels, as shown.

Hold for 30 seconds.

GOAL: To sit on heels with top of feet flat on the floor.

15. Standing Split
(Front, Side and Inverted "Y")

This stretch is for the inner thighs (adductors) and lower back.

Start all three variations by standing with feet as far apart as possible.

FRONT SPLIT:
Bend forward at waist, keeping back straight, head up. Grasp legs with both hands at once.

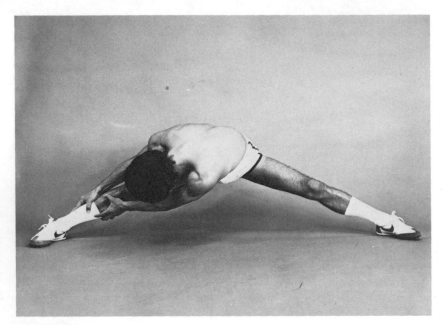

Side Split

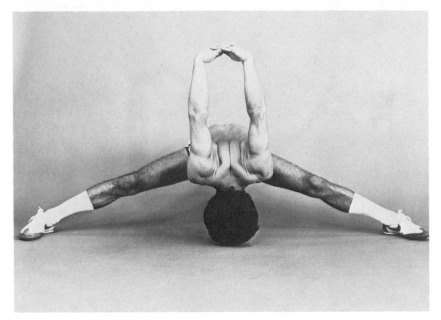

Inverted "Y"

SIDE SPLIT:
Keeping legs spread apart, reach to one side with hands, arms and torso, bringing head toward knee.

INVERTED "Y":
Standing upright with legs apart, clasp hands behind back, and slowly lower head as close to floor as possible. This is an advanced position, so work into it gradually, taking care to hold your balance.

Hold each position for 30 seconds.

GOAL: To hold each stretch at the maximum position possible without losing your balance for 30 seconds.

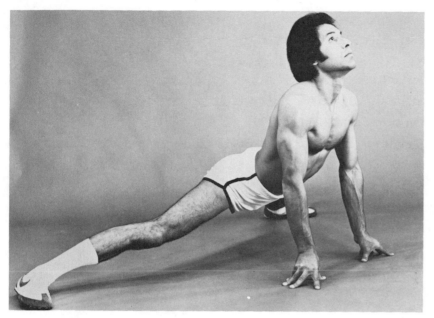

The Cobra

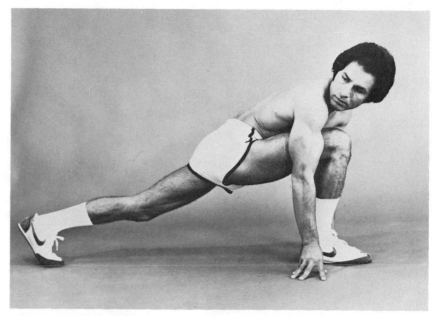

Forward Lunge

16. The Cobra

CAUTION: *If you have a back problem, omit this exercise.*

This stretch is designed primarily to stretch the groin and the inner thighs (adductors).

Spread legs apart as far as possible.

Place hands on floor next to shoulders and lean forward.

Drop the hips as low as possible to the floor and keep the head tilted up.

Hold for 30 seconds.

GOAL: To raise body in position shown, keeping knees and elbows straight.

17. Forward Lunge

This stretch is for the groin and the back of the legs.

Stand straight with feet together.

Lunge forward with left foot, keeping right leg straight.

Left foot should be directly below left knee.

Bring hands to the floor, as shown.

Turn to the left, looking back over your shoulder at your straight leg.

Hold for 30 seconds.

Return to standing position and repeat with right leg forward.

GOAL: To stretch as far down as possible, keeping rear leg straight.

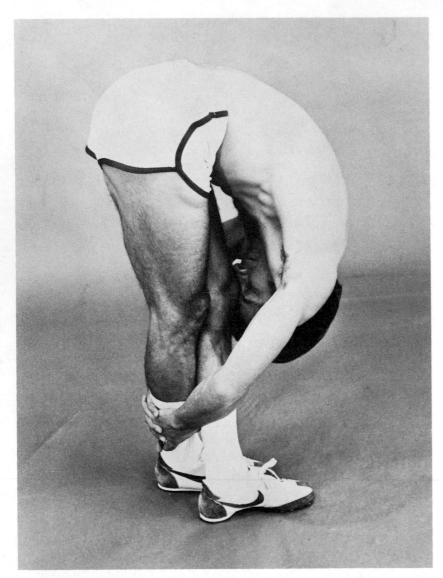

Pretzel Stretch

18. Pretzel Stretch

This stretch is for the back of the thighs (hamstrings) and the lower back.

Stand straight, feet slightly apart, hands at sides.

Cross feet at ankles.

Slowly and gradually, bend forward and clasp hands behind back of legs.

If you lose your balance, place both hands on the floor.

Keep legs straight.

Gently pull head down toward knees.

Hold for 30 seconds without bouncing.

GOAL: To touch forehead to knee while keeping legs straight.

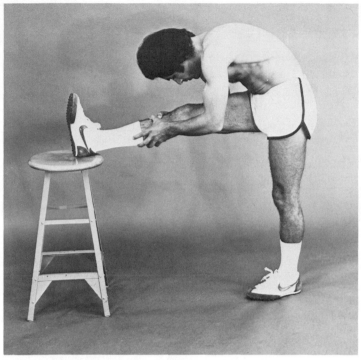

Beginning Ballet Bar Stretch

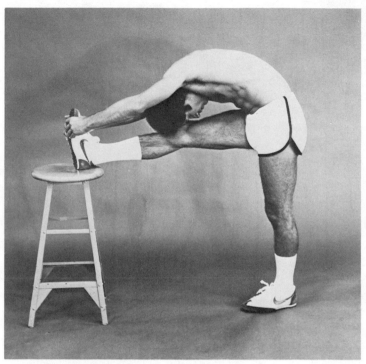

Advanced Ballet Bar Stretch

19. Ballet Bar Stretch
(Beginning and Advanced)

This stretch is for the back of the thighs (hamstrings). (You will need a stool, desk or table on which to rest your foot at a 90° angle.)

Place your left foot on a stable support so that your leg can extend straight out in front of you.

Bend forward, grasping calf with both hands, forehead reaching toward knee.

In advanced position, grasp foot.

Hold for 30 seconds.

Bring extended leg to the floor and repeat with right leg.

GOAL: To hold elevated foot with both hands, keeping the leg straight, and touching forehead to knee.

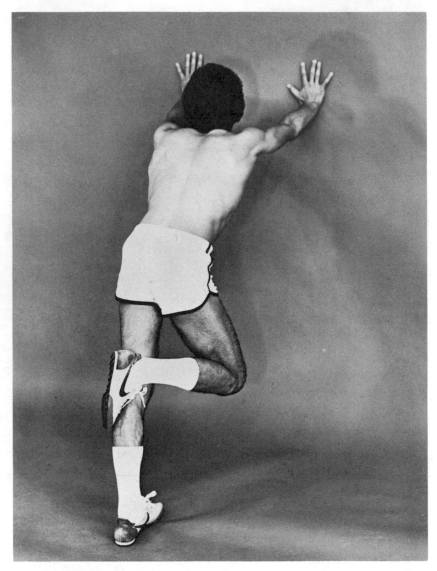

Flying Buttress

20. Flying Buttress

This stretch is for the Achilles tendons and the calf muscles. It is an exercise that is particularly beneficial for tight calf muscles and a good counterbalancing stretch for those who spend a great deal of time in high-heeled shoes.

Stand facing a wall with feet about 3 to 4 feet away.

Lean forward and place both hands against the wall slightly higher than head, as shown.

Place left foot behind right knee.

As you lean forward, keep the heel on the floor, and don't let your buttocks stick out.

Hold for 30 seconds.

Bring left foot to the floor, change sides, and repeat.

GOAL: To lean forward with foot flat on the floor, forming a straight line from back of head to heel.

The Short Stretch

Sitting at a desk all day can produce tension that takes its toll on both mind and body. Make it a regular practice to take a brief mid-day stretch wherever you happen to be at the low point in your day, just to refresh yourself. This is also a useful warm-up routine to accompany your office rope jumping program (detailed in *Chapter 3*).

1. Overhand Stretch

This is one of the easiest and most natural stretches of all.

Clasp your hands in front of you while seated in a chair.

Keeping your fingers together, turn your palms upward toward the ceiling and straighten your arms over your head.

Pull your arms and torso straight up, bend slightly to the left, then slightly to the right.

Hold each position for a few seconds.

Feel the pull through arms, shoulders, back and sides.

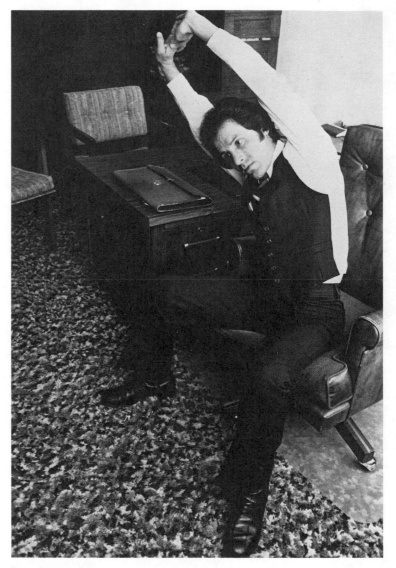

Overhand Stretch

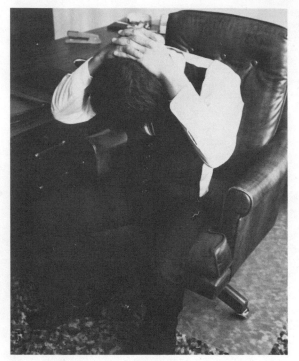

Chin to Chest

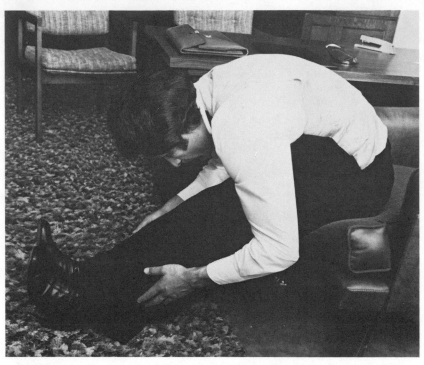

Fold-Over

2. Chin to Chest

This will take the kinks out of your neck and stretch the upper back muscles.

Clasp hands behind your head.

Pull head forward slowly and firmly until chin touches chest.

Hold for 30 seconds and release.

3. Fold-Over

This is an excellent stretch for tired legs and the lower back.

Sit at the edge of your chair.

Extend both legs straight out in front of you, feet dorsiflexed as shown.

Bend forward, grasping calves, ankles or feet with both hands.

Bring forehead as close to knees as possible.

Hold for 30 seconds without bouncing.

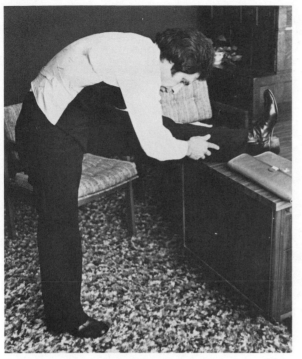

Ballet Bar Stretch (Desk-top Version)

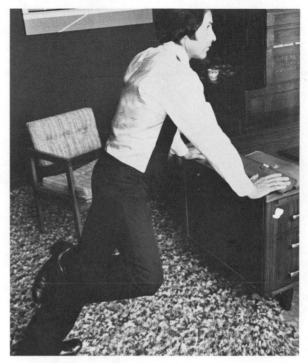

Low Flying Buttress

4. Ballet Bar Stretch *(Desk-top Version)*

This exercise is for the back of the thighs and is identical to the stretch described on page 19.

Place one foot on desk or table.

Keep legs straight and reach forward, bringing forehead as close to knee as possible.

Hold for 30 seconds on each side.

5. Low-Flying Buttress

This is similar to the Flying Buttress described on page 20, with the use of a desk instead of a wall.

Keep heel on the floor and don't let buttocks stick out.

Keep your body as straight as possible from the back of your head to your heel.

Repeat the entire routine or any part of it whenever you need to take a break from stress or tension or to prepare for rope jumping. And, most of all, continue to stretch and enjoy it.

2. PULSE-RATED EXERCISE

The primary purpose of a pulse-rated exercise program is to establish specific performance parameters. Dr. Laurence Morehouse of U.C.L.A. has pointed out that "fitness is not measured in terms of how many pull-ups or sit-ups you can do, or how far you can broad jump, or how fast you can run. Seconds on a stop watch or numbers of repetitions are not equivalent to effort. They tell you nothing about the body's response to the exercise. They don't tell you if you're exercising hard enough, or not hard enough. There's only one way to tell whether you're working at the right intensity and that's by measuring your pulse rate."[1]

Using Pulse Rate to Monitor Your Fitness

There are several areas where the pulsation of the heart can be felt. The radial artery is the most common. If light pressure is applied with both the index and middle fingers, at the position indicated, usually pulsation can be felt.

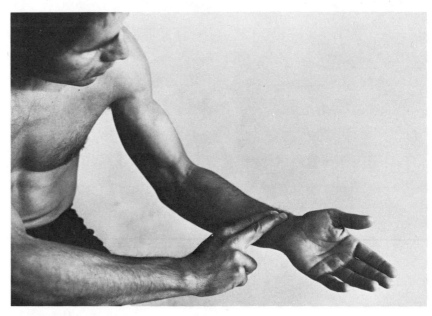

Check pulse rate by applying light pressure to the radial artery, as shown.

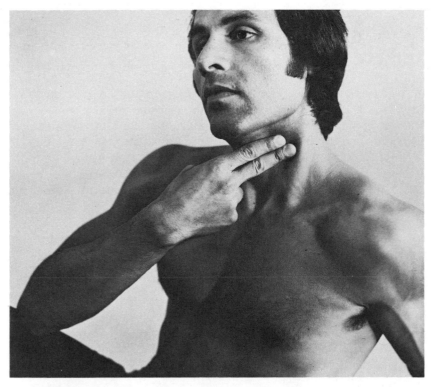

Apply light pressure to the carotid artery in the neck to check pulse rate.

If you have difficulty finding the radial artery, try the carotid artery in the neck. The pulsation there is usually strong and easy to find. Apply light pressure below the lower jaw, but do not compress both sides simultaneously.

Once you locate your pulse, count the beats for ten seconds and multiply by six. This will give you the heart rate for one minute (see Fig. 2-1).

FIG. 2-1
YOUR RESTING HEART RATE

10 Second Count	Heart Rate
8	48
9	54
10	60
11	66
12	72
13	78
14	84
15	90
16	96
17	102
18	108
19	114
20	120
21	126
22	132
23	138
24	144
25	150
26	156
27	162
28	168
29	174
30	180

The list below will give you an idea of normal resting pulse rates, expressed in beats per minutes (BPM). Keep in mind that these are average rates under rest conditions:

Men	72–76 BPM
Women	75–80 BPM
Boys	80–84 BPM
Girls	82–89 BPM

It is not completely understood why women and girls have a slightly higher resting pulse rate than men and boys.

Tachycardia (rapid heartbeat under rest conditions) and bradycardia (slow heartbeat under rest conditions) are terms used to refer to heart rates at either end of the continuum. Tachycardia is a heartbeat over 100 BPM and is undesirable. Bradycardia is a heart rate of less than 60 BPM and is generally considered desirable. A slow heart rate is representative of physical fitness, if it is achieved by exercise. However, it may also be a sign of atrio-ventricular heart block.

Dr. Morehouse points out that the pulse rate changes throughout the day. It is lowest after you have been asleep for about six hours. On awakening it will increase five to ten beats per minute. During the day, the resting pulse rate gradually increases, and at bedtime, it is probably another five to ten beats per minute higher than it was when you got up in the morning.

Pulse rate is one of the best measures of physical fitness. A well-conditioned individual has a slow increase in heart rate upon exercising, and a rapid recovery rate upon termination, whereas an individual in poor condition has a rapid increase in heart rate upon exercising, and a slow, gradual recovery rate upon termination.

Aerobic Exercise and Heart Rate

Activities that increase circulatory-respiratory fitness are called "aerobics." Aerobic exercises include, but are not limited to: rope jumping, running, walking, bicycling, and swimming. By regularly participating in one or more aerobic activities such as these, you can significantly lower your resting pulse rate and decrease the load on your heart. Lowering your resting pulse rate, I might add, is a long-range goal and not something that can be accomplished overnight.

To determine your target heart rate for maximum benefit and safety, start with the number 220 (for males) or 226 (for females), subtract your age, then multiply by 75%. For example, a 40 year old man in average condition would use the following equation: (220 − 40) x 75% = 135 BPM. Two hundred twenty beats per minute minus age is generally regarded as the *maximum* pulse rate for an untrained male and 75% of that is regarded as safe for a male in poor to average condition.

At 135 BPM, this hypothetical average man would be exercising at his *maximum safe* heart rate. At 125 BPM, he would get only 65% of his safe cardiovascular exercise; at 115 BPM, only 20%; and at 105 BPM only 5%. So, at 105 BPM, our average man would have to exercise for 200 minutes, or about 3½ hours, to receive the same exercise as 10 minutes at 135 BPM. This is why it is so very important to exercise at the *highest safe* pulse rate possible.

The "Average Maximal Heart Rates" chart (Fig. 2–2) will allow you to gauge your own target heart rate against averages established by ten European and American investigators. Locate your approximate age first. The first number to the right of age column represents the average maximum heart rate for an individual at a given age. Reading across the column, find the number closest to your actual heart rate during exercise. If you exercise regularly and are in good condition, try to maintain a training pulse rate between 70% and 85% of your maximum heart rate for a minimum of twenty minutes. According to many physiologists, this will give you the ideal training response.

The American Heart Association recommends exercising for a minimum of twenty minutes each day. You can meet this recommendation by supplementing five minutes of rope jumping with fifteen minutes of walking, jogging, cycling, or swimming. Keep in mind the importance of starting out gradually and moderately with whatever you can do comfortably. If you start getting tired, stop and rest. You'll be able to do a little more next time. You'll find that activity sustained during exercise conditions, will eventually produce a decrease in heart rate under rest conditions. Most marathon runners, for example, have resting pulse rates in the forties or fifties. I'm not a marathon runner, but through cardiovascular conditioning, I've been able to lower my resting pulse rate to 42 BPM. You can do the same, and decrease the workload on your heart.

FIG. 2-2

AVERAGE MAXIMAL HEART RATES

Age	Max. H.R.	90% MHR	85% MHR	80% MHR	75% MHR	70% MHR	65% MHR	60% MHR
25	190	171	162	152	143	133	124	114
30	186	167	158	149	140	130	121	112
35	182	164	155	146	137	127	118	109
40	181	163	154	145	136	127	118	109
45	179	161	152	143	134	125	116	107
50	175	158	149	140	131	123	114	105
55	171	154	145	137	128	120	111	103
60	168	151	143	134	126	118	109	101
65	164	148	139	131	123	115	107	98

From the National Workshop on Exercise in the Prevention, in the Evolution, and in the Treatment of Heart Disease, J. S. Carolina Medical Association, Vol. 65, Supplement 1, Dec. 1969.

3. ROPE JUMPING

Why Rope Jumping?

Why not? It's a great cardiovascular exercise! Here are just a few of the advantages:

1. Reduces serum lipids, i.e., cholesterol and triglycerides. Also improves lipoprotein levels (HDL and LDL). These are important because of their relationship to heart disease.

2. Aids in weight loss.

3. Improves stamina and endurance.

4. Reduces resting systolic and diastolic blood pressure.

5. Provides collateral circulation (ingrowth of additional blood vessels). This is of particular importance to someone suffering from atherosclerosis (see *Chapter 6*).

6. Improves balance and coordination.

7. Gets the body into shape for a sport.

8. Trims adipose tissue (fat) off thighs, hips, and legs.

9. Increases maximal oxygen uptake, i.e. it increases the amount of oxygen taken up and utilized by the body.

10. Promotes better sleep.

11. Improve elimination.

12. Provides for mental deceleration, tranquility and peace of mind, or more simply stated, "getting your head together." Psychiatrists have been able to show that people who are depressed become less depressed in response to exercise.

13. Improves sexual performance.

14. Decreases platelet aggregation.[1] In other words, it reduces the clumping together of cells in the arteries. This is desirable because it helps to keep your arteries open.

15. And last but not least, it's fun!

If you haven't checked with your physician, make certain that you do so before you undertake any exercise protocol. If you're over thirty-five and haven't been exercising on a regular basis, I would suggest a stress treadmill test.

Rope Jumping and Cardiovascular Fitness

In the 1960s, Dr. Kaare Rodahl, Director of the Institute of Work Physiology in Oslo, Norway, conducted a research project to test the value of rope jumping. His study was based on a representative sample of American females whose primary exercise consisted of hospital duties, housework and daily walking for short distances.

During the study, the subjects jumped rope for five minutes daily, five times each week for four weeks. When careful measurements of key fitness factors were compared before and after the testing period, those least fit had improved the most, and those most fit had improved the least, but all had improved to some degree.

"During the first week of training," Dr. Rodahl reports, "the mean pulse rate . . . at the fifth minute of rope skipping was 168 BPM. During the last week of training it was 145 BPM."[2] A lowered pulse rate, as you will recall, is an indication of improved endurance.

Dr. Rodahl also measured the pulse rate of a group of similar ages and working conditions who did not jump rope. This control group showed no improvement whatsoever from the beginning to the end of the four-week testing period.

The rope-jumping subjects, by contrast, had increased their average fitness by a statistically significant 25%. These results were particularly noteworthy considering the short duration of each exercise period. Another positive side effect for those who participated in the rope jumping, was that they all experienced some improvement in working efficiency and a reduction of stress-related emotional symptoms.

Dr. Rodahl points out that to build and maintain fitness requires very little time and effort. It is his opinion that, "nothing surpasses the simple jump rope in producing the greatest fitness in the least amount of time."[3] [Italics mine.]

HOW ROPE JUMPING COMPARES TO OTHER ACTIVITIES

In terms of overall exercise for the cardiovascular system, 10 minutes of rope jumping at 120 rotations per minute is equivalent to:

- 30 minutes of jogging (8 minutes per mile)
- 2 sets of singles tennis
- 18 holes of golf
- 2 miles of cycling
- 30 minutes of skiing (snow/water)

At Arizona State University exercise physiologist Jack Baker studied ninety-two students who were out of condition, putting half in a thirty minutes-a-day jogging program, and half in a ten minutes-a-day rope jumping program. When tested, the two groups shared almost identical improvement in cardiovascular efficiency.[4]

COOPER'S AEROBICS POINT SYSTEM

Kenneth Cooper developed a point system by which various aerobic exercises could be comparatively measured.[5] In Cooper's program, the individual accumulates thirty points a week from a selection of activities; each activity has a point value commensurate with its contribution to aerobic fitness. The aerobic point system was derived from laboratory measurements of the oxygen costs of the exercises, as well as data obtained from field tests. The rope jumping point values for both men and women are:

5 minutes	1½ points
10 minutes	3 points
15 minutes	4½ points

Other activities equal to three points are as follows: golf, eighteen holes without motorized cart; jogging, one mile between ten and twelve minutes; cycling, two miles under six minutes or three miles between nine and twelve minutes; swimming, 350 yards between six and nine minutes; handball, squash, and basketball, twenty minutes of continuous play. Thus, rope jumping has a relatively a high aerobics rating in relation to time expended.

As in any exercise, the degree to which fitness is improved is dependent on the way in which the activity is performed. Rope jumping is no exception. Three important factors are: the length of time of each jumping session, the number of rest periods interspersed with jumping, and the rate of rope rotations per minute. Speed, however, is less important than maintaining a consistent rhythm.

WHO SHOULD NOT JUMP ROPE?

You should not jump rope if you have a chronic or acute back condition or if you have any of the following: unstable angina; uncontrolled arrhythmias; uncontrolled diabetes; or signs of circulatory insufficiency such as pallor, diminished pulse, clammy skin, fainting, and incoordination.

Exercise should leave you in a state of relaxation, not create marked or prolonged fatigue. If you are fatigued for longer than two hours following your exercise session, your workout is too strenuous and should be modified.

Individuals of any age, including people over sixty-five, can jump rope—on the condition that they have their doctor's consent and have none of the contraindications mentioned above.

Even if you are in good health, it is always advisable to consult your physician before beginning any exercise program, particularly if it involves a degree of exertion to which you are not accustomed.

The Cause and Cure of Side Stitch

Physicians agree that side stitch is a pain on either side of the abdomen near the rib cage. However, doctors and textbooks do not agree as to what causes a stitch. Some of the possible causes that have been suggested are: (1) faulty breathing techniques; (2) gas in the colon; (3) overeating; (4) weak abdominal muscles; (5) constipation; (6) descended spleen; (7) cramp in the intercostal muscles (muscles between the ribs); (8) spasms of the diaphragm; (9) glycogen depletion of the liver.

However, many rope jumpers and runners who experience side stitch do not have any of these problems, which suggests that these explanations are based on speculation.

Research conducted in New Zealand may offer a more definitive answer to the side stitch controversy. The following is excerpted from the "Executive Fitness Newsletter":

Jack D. Sinclair, professor of physiology at the University of Auckland Medical School, found that side stitch is more common in school children and young athletes than adults. When it does occur in adults it is prevalent in runners, basketball players, soccer and tennis players. Sinclair also noted that jockeys and camel riders sometimes suffer from side stitch. So can people who ride bicycles and motorcycles over bumpy terrain or race boats in rough seas. Pregnant women are also plagued with side stitch. Surprisingly swimmers, rowers and cyclists (on smooth roads) seldom if ever get a pain on the side.

To determine the real cause and cure of side stitch, Professor Sinclair questioned over 100 university athletes. His survey revealed that the most common site of the stitch was the upper right or mid-abdomen region. Some subjects complained of left abdominal pain, but much less frequently. His work showed that the pain occurred many times after heavy eating and drinking and while running downhill or over rough ground. Side stitch appeared more often in a person who was less physically fit.

Deep breathing and bending tended to relieve the pain. Holding the breath when inhaling was also effective, but holding the breath on expiration made the pain worse. Lying on one's back with the hips supported and legs swinging up in the air was another means of alleviating the ache.

These findings led Sinclair to theorize that side stitch is caused by a stretching of the peritoneal ligaments. Attached to and extending from the diaphragm (the huge dome-shaped muscle dividing the chest from the abdomen), these ligaments support the liver, spleen and stomach. Repeated jolts received while running or riding over rough terrain sometimes cause these organs to sag, stretching the peritoneal ligaments. If the abdominal muscles are weak or the stomach is full, tension on the ligaments increases. The peritoneal ligaments pull on the diaphragm, causing the pain we know as side stitch.

Sinclair's theory explains why increased fitness, bending down and postural changes help relieve side stitch. The physically fit person has stronger abdominal muscles which can hold up the body organs and keep the ligaments from stretching out. Bending down or changing posture (as in lying on one's back) allows the ligaments to relax. The pain during expiration and relief on inspiration also fits. When a person inspires, the ligaments collapse, but when he expires they stretch out.

Professor Sinclair's findings were verified by a second researcher, Derek Compton, who did extensive testing with three women and seven men. That report was also published in the New Zealand Journal of Health, Physical Education and Recreation Issue, 1972.[6]

By following some basic rules, you can avoid, or at least reduce this pain:

- Lean forward while sitting and pull your stomach in, attempting to push the abdominal organs up against the diaphragm.
- Lie on your back elevating your legs.
- Avoid holding your breath when exhaling. Hold your breath while inhaling.
- Do not eat 1–2 hours prior to rope jumping or jogging.

What Kind of Clothes Should I Wear?

Wear whatever type of clothing you find most comfortable. During the workday, you can jump rope in whatever you happen to be wearing, although you may want to remove heavy jewelry, jackets or other restrictive items, and change your shoes if they do not have flat soles. Otherwise, if you're in a non-work situation it's more practical to wear a jogging suit, leotards, or shorts and a tank top. I like to let my skin breathe, so jogging shorts and shoes are fine for me. Whatever you do, don't wear any tight clothing. Also, if you perspire considerably, use a couple of wristbands and a head sweatband.

An additional note for women: Experts advise that women participating in sports wear bras, since breast tissue will stretch with continual bouncing.

ARE RUBBERIZED SUITS AND SAUNA SHORTS AND BELTS EFFECTIVE FOR WEIGHT LOSS?

This is a question I'm asked very frequently, and understandably so. Every time you open a magazine or newspaper, you inevitably see an advertisement for sauna belts showing you how to slim your way to slenderness in no time flat, with no effort. Let's examine this question in a little more detail.

The National Athletic Health Institute headed by Dr. Robert Kerlan and Dr. Frank Jobe probably stated it most directly by saying, "Do *not* wear rubberized or plastic clothing while exercising. The increased sweat loss doesn't result in a permanent loss of body weight, and this practice can be very dangerous. The rubberized or plastic clothing doesn't allow the body sweat to evaporate, which is the principal mechanism for temperature regulation in humans during exercise. The result can be a dramatic rise in body temperature, excessive dehydration and salt loss, and eventual heat stroke or heat exhaustion.''[7]

Dr. Marvin M. Lipman and Dr. Harold Aaron, the two principal consultants for Consumer Union's *The Medicine Show*, explain that in recent years there has been a proliferation of wearable products promoted for weight reduction—so-called sauna shorts and belts, body wraps dipped in chemical solutions, and others.[8] All are ineffective at best and some are downright dangerous. Doctors have also warned that body wraps can be hazardous for people suffering from diabetes or diseases of the arteries and veins of the legs.

Dr. Laurence Morehouse explains it this way, ''When you wear rubberized suits, all you're conditioning yourself for is heat acclimatization. When you get such body heat, you can't work hard enough to get into good condition. Rubberized suits may acclimatize you to heat, which is a good idea if you intend to play tennis in the tropics or fight in the desert, but they do absolutely nothing else for you, and they can very well endanger your life.''[9]

I like to explain it this way: the body is 65% water. When you put on a sauna belt, all you're doing is creating a temporary fluid imbalance. It's just like walking into a steam room for a few minutes. Sure, you're going to lose weight because there's going to be a certain amount of fluid loss. However, what most people don't realize is that as soon as you get to the drinking fountain, you'll replenish what you've lost. Save your money.

WHAT TYPE OF FOOT ATTIRE IS BEST FOR ROPE JUMPING?

Running shoes are best for rope jumping. There are a wide variety of running shoes available. Look for those with good absorbency and padding. When trying on new shoes, always take the measurements standing and near the end of the day when your feet are slightly larger. The shoe will then accommodate for foot swelling. If you have no choice, pick a shoe that's a little on the large side rather than one that is too small, particularly if you have Morton's Syndrome (a long second toe). Also, it's wise to wear cotton socks for rope jumping and running. Cotton absorbs perspiration and adds cushioning, while nylon and other synthetic materials retain heat and moisture.

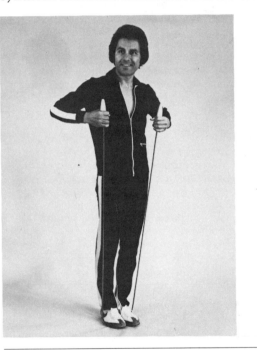

HOW TO SELECT THE RIGHT ROPE

Stand on the middle of the rope—the handles should reach the underarms. If the rope is too long for you, tie a knot near one or both handles. Remember, you can always take a long rope and make it shorter, but you can't take a short rope and make it longer. If in doubt, try the rope out in the store.

Do's and Don'ts for Rope Jumping

DO stretch before you begin any exercise. (see *Chapter 3.*)

DO jump in front of a mirror so you can observe what you're doing, particularly in the beginning.

DO bend your knees slightly.

DO use your wrists for more effective rope contol.

DO jump on a soft surface such as a wooden floor, rug, or grass, whenever possible.

DO be patient with yourself and don't get discouraged if you can't master the rope immediately. It takes most people about two weeks to master the basics.

DO keep your legs in front of your body—never behind. If you jump with your legs up behind you, the rope may tangle with your ankles. It will also fatigue you sooner and create a temporary postural imbalance while jumping.

DO make rope jumping an enjoyable experience. Jump to your favorite music, be it classical, jazz or disco.

DON'T look down at the rope; look straight ahead.

DON'T jump too high. The mistake most people make is to jump too high and land too hard, increasing the amount of shock and trauma to the joints and lower back. You only need to jump about one inch off the ground. Jump on the balls of the feet and "think light," i.e., don't allow your feet to come slamming down.

DON'T jump with bare feet. (See Proper Foot Attire, p. 32.)

DON'T hold your hands in too close or too far away. The correct position is with your elbows slightly bent, upper arms in, and hands held about a foot from the hips. (See Starting Position, p. 34.)

DON'T allow the rope to slap the floor. It should skim the surface slightly.

DON'T let "wobbles" get into the rope as it turns. If you do, this indicates insufficient control.

DON'T EVER stand still after you finish rope jumping, as this will tend to pool blood away from the heart. Blood pooling in the lower extremities may drop your blood pressure and result in subsequent faintness. Lie down, sit, or walk around.

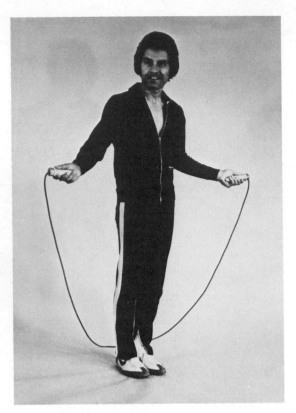

Starting Position

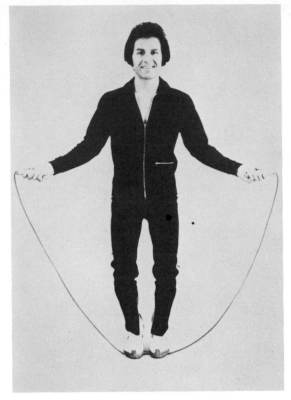

Basic Jump

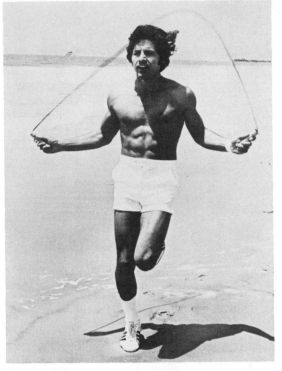

Jogging while jumping rope is not a difficult skill to learn and results in less stress on the body than jumping in place. *Photo by Erik Stern.*

The Basic Jump

Stand with feet about two to three inches apart.

Keep knees slightly bent, weight on the balls of the feet.

Look straight ahead, not down.

Rotate the rope making small circles with the wrists and lower arms.

Jump only about one inch off the ground with each rotation.

Jump and Jog

All weight-bearing exercises such as running in place and rope jumping produce some shock and trauma. By adding forward movement, this stress is minimized. Practice moving around when you jump rope as opposed to always jumping in place. With a little more work, you can learn to jog and jump rope simultaneously.

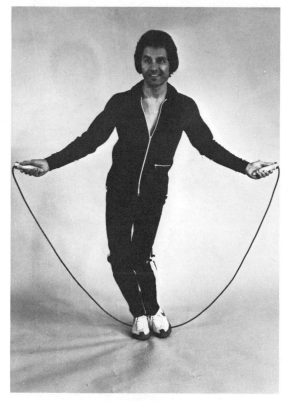

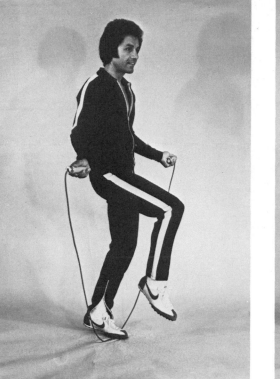

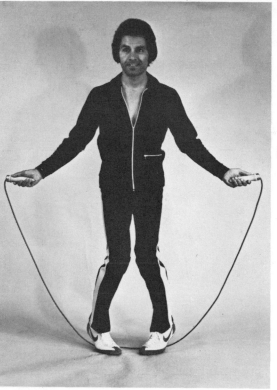

Side-to-Side—good exercise for skiers.

One-Leg Jump

Toes In: Step 1

Beginning Variations

Rope Jumping Variations

After you have mastered the basic jump, you may want to try some of the variations shown here.

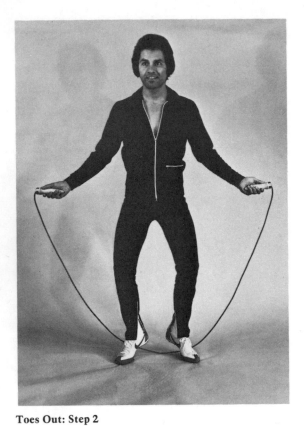

Toes Out: Step 2

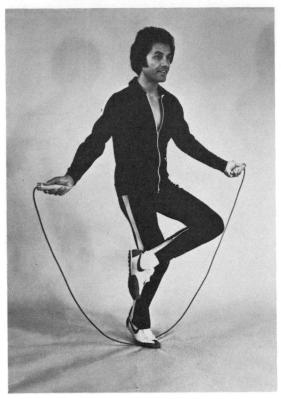

Leg Cross

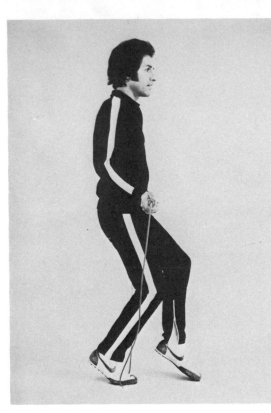

Anterior Toe Tap: Step 1

Intermediate Variations

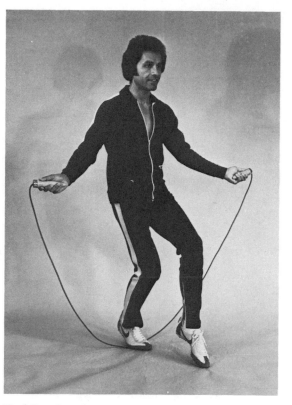

Posterior Toe Tap: Step 2

Heel-Toe: Step 1

Heel-Toe: Step 2

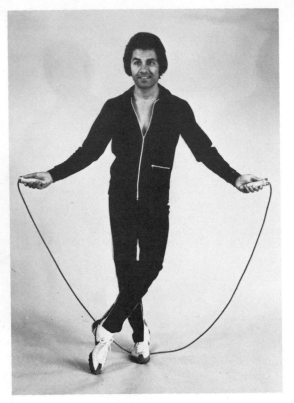

Anterior-Lateral Toe Tap: Step 1

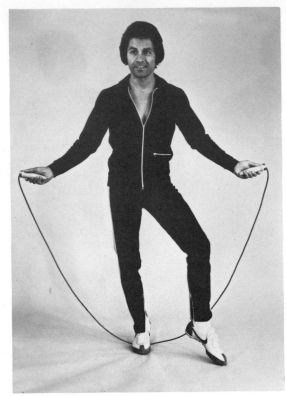

Anterior-Lateral Toe Tap: Step 2

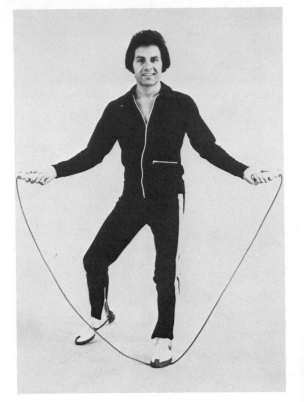

Posterior-Lateral Toe Tap: Step 1

38

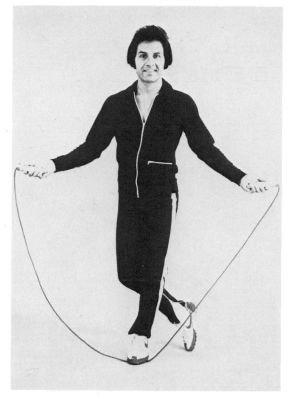

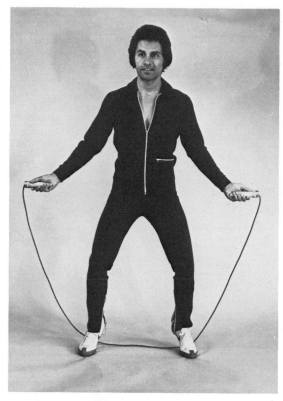

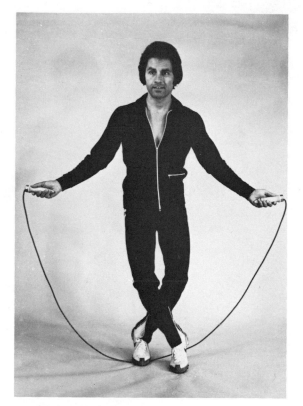

Posterior-Lateral Toe Tap: Step 2

Straddle Crossover: Step 1

Straddle Crossover: Step 2

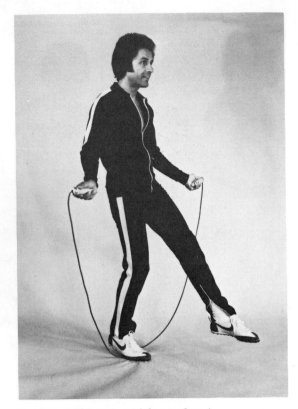

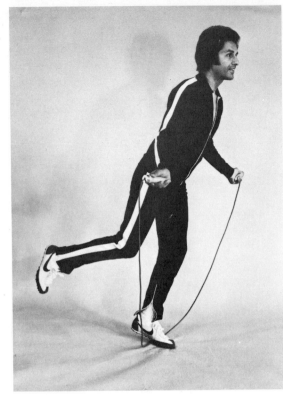

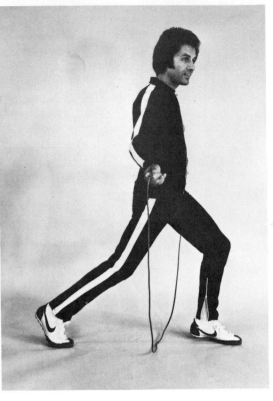

Anterior Alternate Leg Kickouts: Step 1   **Posterior Alternate Leg Kickouts: Step 2**   Lunges

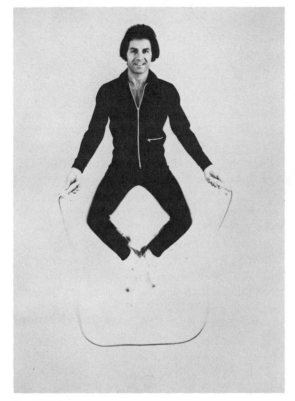

Heel Clicks

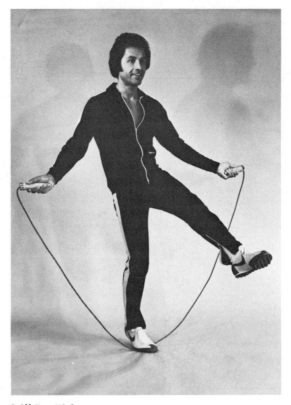

Stiff-Leg Kickouts

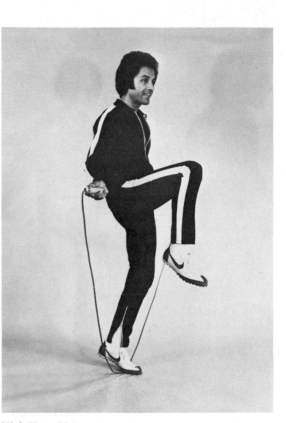

High-Knee Kicks

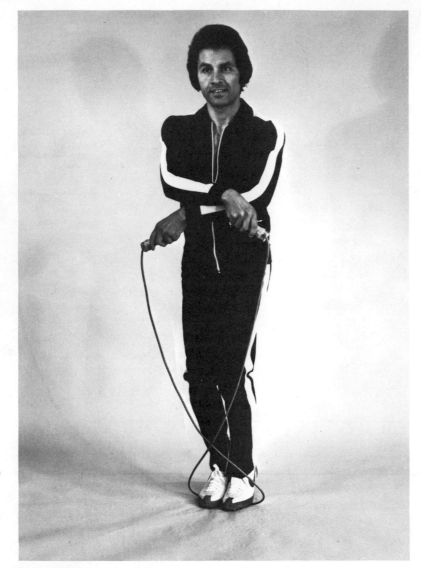

The Luna Loop

Advanced and Expert Variations

The Luna Loop

Start with the basic jump.

Cross arms in front and jump over rope.

Uncross arms and jump again.

Tilt wrists down slightly.

CAUTION: Cross arms far enough across chest to allow room to jump through.

ADVANCED VARIATIONS:

Hold crossover while jumping.

Hold crossover while jogging.

Stiff-leg kickouts with crossover.

EXPERT VARIATION: Crossover and open in one jump.

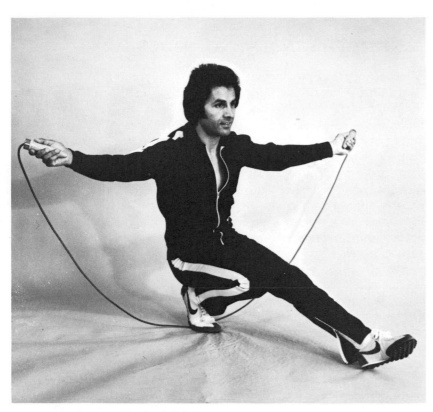

Russian Kickouts—not for bad knees.

Establishing a Routine

WHEN SHOULD I JUMP ROPE AND HOW OFTEN?

There is no such thing as a "best time" to exercise. It's all based on individual preference. Some people function much better in the morning, while with others, it's just the opposite. Most people can easily adjust their exercise sessions to their daily schedules. The important thing is that you exercise at least three to five times per week.

A word of advice for those who live in hot climates: It takes energy to lose heat. This energy comes from the activity of your sudoriferous (sweat) glands. These glands, and there are millions of them, use metabolic energy to secrete perspiration. In attempting to maintain a normal body temperature, energy that you could be using more productively is drained and depleted. This is one reason why people fatigue so easily on a hot day. So, to use the energy more effectively in a hot climate, exercise either early in the morning, or after the sun has gone down, or, of course, in a cool building. It's also a good idea to wait one to two hours after a meal before exercising.

HOW LONG SHOULD I JUMP?

Jump rope for a minimum of five minutes per day—however, don't begin by jumping that long. Concentrate on the mechanics first, such as bending your knees and coming down on the balls of your feet. If you've never jumped rope before, start out by practicing *without* the rope in front of a mirror until you master the basics. Once you've accomplished this, introduce the rope and start out slowly and comfortably until you can gradually work up to five minutes non-stop.

Many people overexert and attempt to go beyond their capacity. *Listen to your body and pay attention to its signals.* Check your pulse from time to time to make sure you're within your target heart rate.

Following is a suggested eight-week progressive schedule for rope jumping (Fig. 3–1) that will help you build up to five minutes of rope jumping per day and add jumping variations over a period of eight weeks. Whether you are at the beginning, intermediate, advanced, or expert level, always stretch prior to rope jumping.

Again, I recommend that you include other activities such as jogging, swimming, tennis, racquetball, or weight training in conjunction with your five minutes of rope jumping to develop a well-rounded exercise program.

FIG. 3–1
EIGHT-WEEK PROGRESSIVE SCHEDULE

Week	Minutes	Number of Jumps	Variations
One	1	50–100	Basic Jump only
Two	2	100–200	Basic Jump only
Three	3	200–300	Basic Jump only
Four	4	300–400	Basic Jump only
Five	5	400–500	Beginning variations
Six	5	500–600	Beginning variations
Seven	5	500–600	Beginning and Intermediate variations
Eight	5	500–600	Beginning, Intermediate and Advanced variations

PAUL SMITH'S ENDURANCE PROGRAM

Another way to approach your rope jumping program is through Paul Smith's endurance program (Fig. 3–2). Paul Smith is Coordinator of Health, Physical Education and Athletics for the Shoreline School, District of Seattle, Washington, as well as author of the book, *Rope Skipping: Rhythms, Routines, Rhymes.* Smith's program is based on interval training, which is currently being used very successfully by the East Germans. Interval training consists of short, intensive bouts of exercise along with equally short rest periods. At Level One, you would jump for fifteen seconds, then rest for fifteen seconds, repeating this procedure four times for a total of one minute of exercise. At each succeeding level, the length of the exercise bout is increased and the length of the rest perod decreased until, by Level Eighteen, you are able to rope jump continuously for eighteen minutes.

If you decide to attempt this program—and I hope you will —*do not* try to go all out initially to prove to yourself what great shape you're in. Start out at Level One and gradually move on to each level as you feel ready. It may take you several weeks or months, but when you finally reach eighteen minutes of nonstop jumping, you will feel a tremendous sense of accomplishment. When I first started out several years ago, I used to huff and puff through fifty jumps. I felt awkward and clumsy. Only recently, I jumped 10,000 consecutive times in one hour and fifteen minutes. By gradually increasing your endurance, you can do the same, and even better.

FIG. 3–2

THE PAUL SMITH ENDURANCE PROGRAM

Level No.	Turns per minute	Length of Exercise Bout	Length of Rest Period	Repetition of Exercise Bout	Frequency per week	Total Time Rope Jumping Daily
1	60	15 sec.	15 sec.	4	5	1.0 min.
2	60	15 sec.	15 sec.	6	5	1.5 min.
3	60	30 sec.	15 sec.	4	5	2.0 min.
4	60	30 sec.	15 sec.	6	5	3.0 min.
5	60	45 sec.	15 sec.	4	5	3.0 min.
6	60	45 sec.	15 sec.	6	5	4.5 min.
7	60	1.0 min.	30 sec.	6	5	6.0 min.
8	60	1.5 min.	30 sec.	6	5	9.0 min.
9	60	2.0 min.	1 min.	6	5	12.0 min.
10	60	2.5 min.	1 min.	5	5	12.5 min.
11	60	2.5 min.	1 min.	6	5	15.0 min.
12	60	3.0 min.	1 min.	6	5	18.0 min.
13	60	4.0 min.	1 min.	5	3–5	20.0 min.
14	60	6.0 min.	1 min.	3	3–5	18.0 min.
15	60	9.0 min.	1 min.	2	3–5	18.0 min.
16	60	14.0 min.	0 min.	1	3–5	14.0 min.
17	60	16.0 min.	0 min.	1	3–5	16.0 min.
18	60	18.0 min.	0 min.	1	3–5	18.0 min.

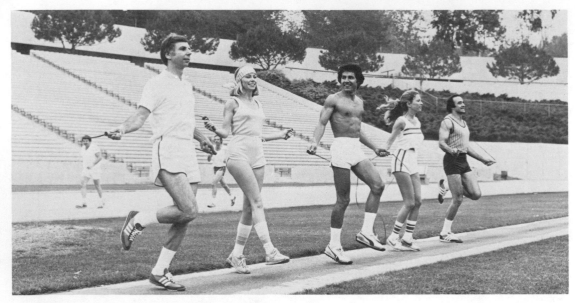

Jump rope with a group or class to keep your interest level high, but compete only with yourself.
Photo by Layne of L.A.

How Can I Keep Up My Interest in Rope Jumping?

Most people start an exercise program with a lot of enthusiasm, and after a short period of time interest begins to wane. Keep in mind that a fitness program should be a lifetime pursuit. Dr. George Sheehan, a prominent New Jersey cardiologist, points out that the reason fitness programs fail is because of the forces behind our contemporary lifestyles. Our culture is a knowledge-oriented culture that tends to regard the body as a second-class citizen. Unless we begin to think of it otherwise, Sheehan feels —and I agree—your fitness program will fail. The following are a few suggestions for keeping your interest up:

1. Either select activities you enjoy, or learn to enjoy the activities in which you participate.

2. Jump rope at a regular time of the day, and make this a part of your daily routine.

3. Jump rope and exercise with a partner, or in a class or group. However, don't get talked into competition. If you do compete, compete only with yourself.

4. Jump rope to music.

5. Set goals for yourself. Your goal might be to master as many of the rope jumping combinations as possible, or to work up to 500 jumps in succession without missing.

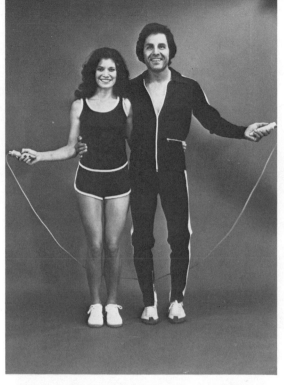

Side by Side—Hold on to each other's waists and jump together.

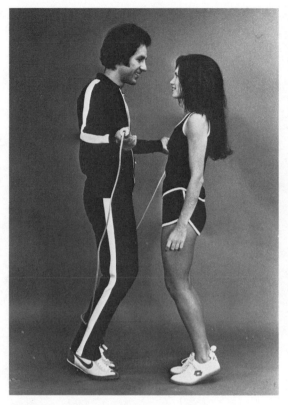

Face to Face—One person turns the rope, while both jump.

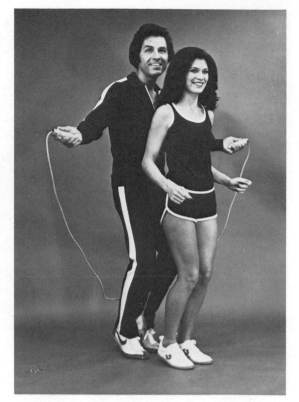

Tandem—One person stands behind the other and turns rope, while both jump.

DOUBLES JUMPING

Jumping rope with another person can be both fun and challenging. Synchronize the rotation of the rope and become doubles champions!

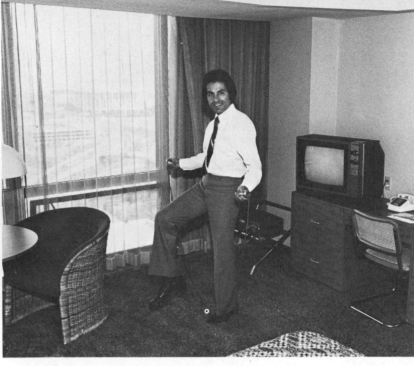

Take your jump rope on a business trip or vacation and exercise in your hotel room.

YOU CAN TAKE IT WITH YOU

The only thing you really need for rope jumping is the rope itself. So why not take it along and exercise wherever you happen to be—in your office, hotel room, at the track or on the beach, not to mention your own living room. If the rope touches the ceiling, simply tie a knot or two at the ends, and go for it!

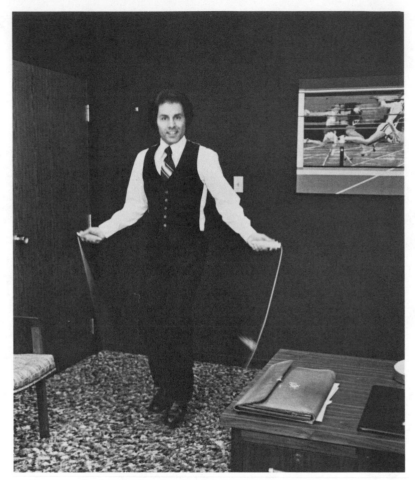

Make your coffee break a jumping break.

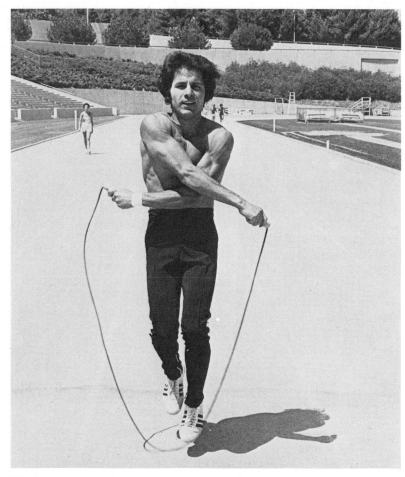

The Luna Loop on the track. Many runners also jump rope inside during bad weather to stay in shape.
Photo by Erik Stern.

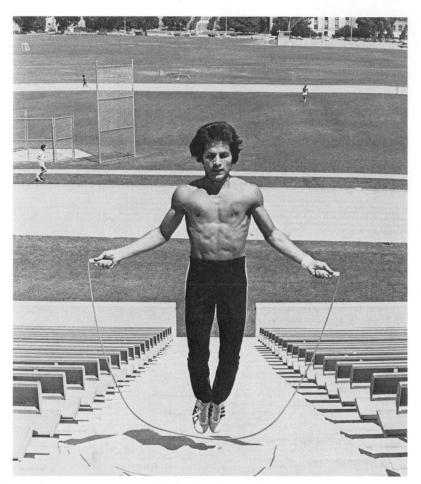

Jumping rope up steps. This is for advanced rope jumpers only.
Photo by Erik Stern.

World Records for Rope Jumping

In rope jumping, as in many other physical activities, attempts have been made to establish world records. The following outstanding performances are from the *Guinness Book of World Records* for 1977:[10]

- Greatest number of turns ever performed without a break or fault:
  50,000 in 5 hours, 15 minutes.
  Rabbi Barry Silberg
  Milwaukee, Wisconsin
  May, 1976

- Most turns in one jump: 5
  Katsumi Suzuki
  Tokyo, Japan
  1968

- Most turns in one minute: 286
  J. Rogers
  Melbourne, Australia
  November 10, 1937
    and
  T. Lewis
  Melbourne, Australia
  September 16, 1939

- Most turns in ten seconds: 57
  LuAnn Stolt
  Bloomer, Wisconsin
  1972

- Most double turns: 2,736
  Kaori Sumitani
  Tokyo, Japan
  April 14, 1976

- Most triple turns: 110
  Katsumi Suzuki
  Tokyo, Japan
  November 28, 1975

- Longest distance jumped:
  1,264 miles from Brisbane to Cairns, Australia
  Tom Morris
  1963

4. THE SENSIBLE DIET

A Long-Range Program for Better Nutrition

We live in a land of overabundance, and, in the area of health, "more" often means "less." It is becoming increasingly evident that the air we breathe contains more than just air, the water we drink contains more than just water, and the foods we eat contain more than just nutrients. No wonder we often get discouraged.

Dr. William Glasser, author of *Positive Addiction*, writes, "The simple statement we sometimes say out loud but more often say to ourselves: 'The hell with it,' means we are settling for less because we don't have it in us now to struggle for more. We settle for less with our marriages, our children, our employers, and our neighbors than we know we should. We drink, we smoke, we eat too much and too many of the wrong kinds of foods because it's easier than disciplining ourselves to say no. I am not recommending that we should be more rigid or contentious, for that too, is weakness. It takes strength, however, to be warm, firm, humorous, and caring and still do what we know we ought to do. Our lives would be much better if we never said, 'The hell with it.' "[1]

Getting people to change their eating habits is a very difficult task. It's much easier to say, "The hell with it!" But we may not be able to go on saying that indefinitely. Many people come to me seeking help. Many of them are walking time bombs. After years of apathy, indifference, abuse, and neglect, some have become heart attack or stroke victims. Others are suffering from acute pain in their backs or joints, most having waited until a catastrophe befell them before they realized that some changes had to be made.

By practicing preventative medicine and becoming "positively addicted" to exercise and good nutrition, you lower the risk factors against you and improve the quality of your life. By eating sensibly, you increase your level of resistance.

Dr. Paavo Airola, President of the International Academy of Biological Medine, defines the fundamental cause of disease in this manner: "The basic premise of Biological Medicine is that most diseases have the same basic underlying causes. These are: the systemic derangement and biochemical and metabolic disorder brought about by prolonged physical and mental stresses to which the patient has been subjected—such as faulty nutritional patterns, constant overeating, overindulgence in proteins, fats, or refined sugars, nutritional deficiencies, sluggish metabolism and consequent retention of toxic metabolic wastes, exogenous poisons from polluted food, water, air, and environment, toxic drugs, tobacco and alcohol, lack of sufficient exercise, rest and relaxation, and severe emotional and physical stresses. These health-destroying environmental factors bring about derangement in all vital body functions with consequent biochemical imbalance in the tissues, autotoxemia, chronic undersupply of oxygen to the cells, poor digestion, ineffective assimilation of nutrients, and gradually *lower resistance to disease*. Thus, Biological Medicine considers not the bacteria, but the *weakened organism or the lowered resistance* as the primary cause of disease.''[2]

Bacteria are always present in our environment. They are under control if we maintain our natural health and natural resistance. This, unfortunately, is where most of us fail, and when we do, the bacteria are ready to step in and do damage as soon as the resistance is lowered.

The Sensible Diet presented here is a broad, preventative nutritional plan, designed as a guideline for establishing and improving eating patterns. Don't think of it in terms of what you will have to give up, but rather of what you will gain from better dietary habits. Whether your dietary modifications are on a large or small scale will depend on your present patterns. Basically, all you will be doing is eliminating those foods which don't have any nutritional value or very little nutritional value, and replacing them with foods that are vital and nutritious.

The Sensible Diet will also help you reduce some of the risk factors in such degenerative diseases as heart disease, diabetes, cerebral vascular disease (stroke), and certain forms of arthritis.

The Sensible Diet with its emphasis on high complex carbohydrates can be used for weight loss. However, keep in mind that to lose weight, your energy expenditure must be greater than your intake. Here's where regular exercise will play an important role. If intake is the same as output, weight remains the same. And, of course, we all know that if intake is greater than output, weight increases.

However, the primary reason for the Sensible Diet is to prevent what I refer to as the "yo-yo syndrome." Most of the people that I've counseled over the years have gone from one dietary protocol to another without success. Many go through an entire lifetime seeking the "ideal diet" even though there is no such thing. So what happens? You optimistically launch yourself into some popular and well-recommended diet. You feel very self-righteous for a few weeks as you see your weight start to drop. Then, after you've lost as much as you need, you let the diet fall by the wayside, only to put the pounds right back on again in less time than it took to lose them. It doesn't matter which diet is followed. The pattern remains the same, and for good reason: How long can you eat only cottage cheese, lettuce and alfalfa sprouts? How long can you stick to a 500 k calorie a day diet with weekly injections? How long are you going to keep track of the number of carbohydrates you consume per day? How long are you going to exist on appetite suppressants and water pills? Losing the weight is not what's difficult; the hard part is *keeping the weight off*. And that can only be done with sensible and practical dietary intervention.

The Sensible Diet is designed with just this in mind—to help you prevent the "yo-yo" syndrome. It was developed to help you establish a lifelong dietary pattern based on systematic undereating with a recommended weight loss of approximately one to two pounds per week, *but not more*. There's no need to rush—it took you a long time to put the weight on, so don't try to take it off overnight.

Even if your goal is not to lose weight, but simply to stay fit, the Sensible Diet will provide the basis for sound nutrition that can be maintained for a lifetime. The Sensible Diet is an attempt to provide you with the best dietary information currently available. It includes a list of foods that are recommended, a discussion of those items to avoid, a sample menu plan and selected recipes.

Each week, if you so desire, you can have one splurge of

your favorite fat-filled, high-cholesterol, sugar-laden or chemical-laced foods. You decide what that splurge will be. This occasional reprieve will serve to eliminate any feelings of deprivation or depression that often accompany a major change in eating habits. After a while, you may find, to your surprise, that the junk foods you once relished are no longer as desirable.

Work into these healthful eating habits gradually in order to adapt them to your own individual needs. Don't try to make too many changes at once. Remember, your goal is to make the Sensible Diet a lifelong habit.

Recommended Foods

The foods below are recommended, with the reservations indicated. Taken together, they form the basis for the Sensible Diet. They are: (1) low-fat dairy products; (2) limited amounts of fish and poultry; (3) a wide variety of vegetables and fruits; (4) whole grain breads and cereals, especially those with high fiber content; and (5) selected nuts and seeds.

DAIRY PRODUCTS

Low-fat or non-fat milk
Low-fat cottage cheese
Low-fat plain yogurt (not fruit flavored)
Cheese (skim or low-fat)
3–5 eggs per week, maximum

FISH & POULTRY

Saltwater fish: Limit to once per week. Much of the water in our rivers and lakes is exposed to high levels of toxicity, industrial waste, lead, and mercury. Pollution in the oceans is rapidly equaling that of our fresh waters.

Poultry: Limit to once per week. Hormones and antibiotics are often used in the raising of poultry. This has been associated with a high incidence of chicken leukosis (cancerous tumors). Unfortunately, these tumors are often cut out and the remaining poultry is sold as chicken parts to your local supermarket or grocery store. Even though most commercially grown poultry is fine, it's difficult to determine which has been contaminated or infected by disease.

VEGETABLES

Choose widely from the list below, selecting a variety of green, yellow and leafy vegetables.

Alfalfa sprouts	Cucumbers
Artichokes	Green peppers
Asparagus	Jicama
Beans	Lettuce (Romaine)
Bean sprouts	Mushrooms
Broccoli	Potatoes (include skin)
Brussels sprouts	Pumpkin
Cabbage	Squash
Carrots	Tomatoes
Collard greens	Turnip greens
Corn	Yams

The following vegetables are high in oxalic acid, and should be eaten in limited quantities or with other foods: beet greens; rhubarb; spinach; and Swiss chard.

FRUITS

If you don't need to lose weight, eat as many fresh fruits as you like. Otherwise, limit your intake of fruits to no more than

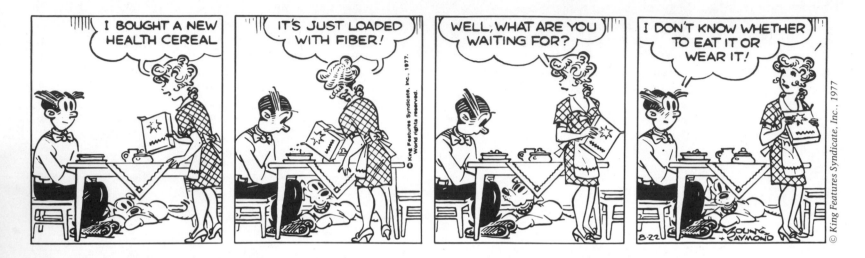

three a day. Avoid canned fruits. I recommend one 8 oz. glass of citrus juice (orange or grapefruit), pineapple or tomato juice, and two pieces of fresh fruit per day.

BREADS, CEREALS AND HIGH FIBER FOODS

Breads should be either dark or brown. Natural grain cereals such as rolled oats and cracked wheat which may be purchased in a health food store are recommended. The following commercial cereals are also recommended: Quick Quaker Oats, Post Grapenuts, Nabisco Shredded Wheat, and Quaker Whole Wheat Hot Natural Cereal. Most other commercially packaged breakfast cereals probably have more nutritional value in the box than the contents. Make it a habit to read labels. If the cereal product contains white or brown sugar, turbinado sugar, molasses, syrups or artificial sweeteners, leave it on the shelf.

Include high fiber foods such as natural cereals and dark or brown breads. A high fiber diet is one containing approximately thirteen grams or more of crude fiber, while a restricted fiber diet is one containing three to five grams. The daily adult requirement for fiber is six grams per day. Dietary fiber increases stool frequency and decreases transit time. Lack of roughage has been linked to heart disease, cancer of the colon, gallstones, diabetes, hiatus hernias, hemorrhoids, appendicitis and diverticulitis.

One of the questions I am most frequently asked, and understandably so, is "What do you recommend for constipation?" The average person in the United States has a bowel movement about once every two days. Whereas in Africa, for example, the Bantus and the Masai have two or three bowel movements in one day. The difference, according to some authorities, lies in the consumption of dietary fiber and the underconsumption of refined foods in these cultures, along with higher levels of activity.

Chronic constipation is generally due to lack of dietary fiber. One of the best sources of fiber is bran, preferably Miller's Bran, which you can purchase at any health food store. (See Fig.

4–1.) I don't recommend the commercial 100% bran cereals because of some of the ingredients they contain. Instead, take a tablespoon of Miller's Bran and sprinkle it into a salad or a bowl of cereal.

Additional causes of chronic constipation are insufficient water; constant worry and tension; too many over-refined foods, or too much animal protein; postponement of bowel movements, which, incidentally, is one of the principal causes of hemorrhoids; and, of course, lack of exercise which stimulates peristalsis (progressive, wormlike movement of food in the intestinal tract). It is reported that on a high fiber diet, food passes through the gastrointestinal tract in thirty to thirty-six hours, while on a low-fiber diet, it takes more than eighty hours.

FIG. 4–1

Sources of Fiber	Percentage of Crude Fiber
Bran (preferably Miller's bran)	9.0%
Dry beans, lentils	4.0%
Nuts	2.5%
Whole wheat bread	1.6%
White bread	.2%
Oatmeal	1.3%
Brown rice	.9%
White rice	.3%
Whole orange	.5%
Orange juice	.1%
Apple	1.0%
Apple sauce	.6%
Apple juice	Trace

Dr. Denis P. Burkitt, one of the leading researchers of dietary fiber, has indicated that one manner of determining whether or not you're getting enough dietary fiber is by examining your stool. If the stool floats in the water, you're consuming enough fiber. However, if the stool sinks, you are advised to increase your fiber consumption.

NUTS AND SEEDS

Eat nuts and seeds with moderation because of their high fat content. Almonds, filberts, sunflower and pumpkin seeds are best. Buy only those that are unsalted and unprocessed.

Items to Avoid

The following food items should be avoided or eliminated entirely from the diet, with allowances, of course, for the occasional splurge. The items to avoid are: refined or simple carbohydrates, red meats, excessive salt, saturated fats, soft drinks, alcoholic beverages, coffee and tea, canned and preserved foods, and high-cholesterol foods.

REFINED OR SIMPLE CARBOHYDRATES

Avoid all white sugar, brown sugar, raw sugar, turbinado sugar, honey, molasses, syrups, dextrose, and artificial sweeteners. The average American consumes 125 pounds of sugar per year. (See Fig. 4–2.) Let the natural sugars in fruit satisfy the desire for sweets.

FIG. 4–2

"HIDDEN SUGARS" IN FOODS

Food Item	Size Portion	Approximate sugar content in teaspoonfuls of granulated sugar
BEVERAGES		
Cola drinks	1 (6 oz. glass)	3½
Cordials	1 (¾ oz. glass)	1½
Ginger ale	6 oz.	5
Hi-ball	1 (6 oz. glass)	2½
Orange-ade	1 (8 oz. glass)	5
Root beer	1 (10 oz. bottle)	4½
Seven-up	1 (6 oz. glass)	3¾
Soda pop	1 (8 oz. bottle)	5
Sweet cider	1 cup	6
Whiskey sour	1 (3 oz. glass)	1½
CAKES & COOKIES		
Angel food	1 (4 oz. piece)	7
Applesauce cake	1 (4 oz. piece)	5½
Banana cake	1 (2 oz. piece)	2
Cheesecake	1 (4 oz. piece)	2
Chocolate cake (plain)	1 (4 oz. piece)	6
Chocolate cake (Iced)	1 (4 oz. piece)	10
Coffeecake	1 (4 oz. piece)	4½
Cupcake (iced)	1	6
Fruit cake	1 (4 oz. piece)	5
Jelly-roll	1 (2 oz. piece)	2½
Orange cake	1 (4 oz. piece)	4
Pound cake	1 (4 oz. piece)	5

Food Item	Size Portion	Approximate sugar content in teaspoonfuls of granulated sugar
Sponge cake	1 (1 oz. piece)	2
Strawberry shortcake	1 serving	4
Brownies (unfrosted)	1 (¾ oz.)	3
Chocolate cookies	1	1½
Fig newtons	1	5
Ginger snaps	1	3
Macaroons	1	6
Nut cookies	1	1½
Oatmeal cookies	1	2
Sugar cookies	1	1½
Chocolate eclair	1	7
Cream puff	1	2
Donut (plain)	1	3
Donut (glazed)	1	6
Snail	1 (4 oz. piece)	4½
CANDIES		
Average milk chocolate bar	1 (1½ oz.)	2½
Chewing gum	1 stick	½
Chocolate cream	1 piece	2
Butterscotch chew	1 piece	1
Chocolate mints	1 piece	2
Fudge	1 oz. square	4½
Gum drop	1	2
Hard candy	4 oz.	20
Lifesavers	1	½
Peanut brittle	1 oz.	3½

Food Item	Size Portion	Approximate sugar content in teaspoonsuls of granulated sugar
CANNED FRUITS & JUICES		
Canned apricots	4 halves with syrup	3½
Canned fruit juices (sweetened)	½ cup	2
Canned peaches	2 halves with syrup	3½
Fruit salad	½ cup	3½
Fruit syrup	2 Tbsp.	2½
Stewed fruits	½ cup	2
DAIRY PRODUCTS		
Ice cream	⅓ pt. (3½ oz.)	3½
Ice cream bar	1	1–7
Ice cream cone	1	3½
Ice cream soda	1	5
Ice cream sundae	1	7
Malted milk shake	1 (10 oz. glass)	5
JAM & JELLIES		
Apple butter	1 Tbsp.	1
Jelly	1 Tbsp.	1–1½
Orange marmalade	1 Tbsp.	1–1½
Peach butter	1 Tbsp.	1
Strawberry jam	1 Tbsp.	1–1½

Food Item	Size Portion	Approximate sugar content in teaspoonsuls of granulated sugar
DESSERTS, MISCELLANEOUS		
Apple cobbler	½ cup	3
Blueberry cobbler	½ cup	3
Custard	½ cup	2
French pastry	1 (4 oz. piece)	5
Jello	½ cup	4½

Reprinted with permission from Dr. Kurt W. Donsbach, copyright 1975

Nathan Pritikin of the Longevity Center in Santa Monica points out that, "Table sugar, honey, molasses, and so forth have the property of increasing blood fats (triglycerides) and increasing the clinical signs of diabetes. Diabetes and atherosclerosis are related because they're caused by certain of the same dietary elements. In addition, a person who has diabetes is very likely to develop atherosclerosis and vice versa."[3]

Dr. Thomas Jukes, University of California at Berkeley, points out in a recent article on sugar that, "Those who say white sugar is bad, but brown sugar good and honey even better, are mistaken. Brown sugar is basically sucrose coated with molasses. Honey has a different makeup, but the amount of vitamins and minerals it supplies is negligible. Nutritionally speaking, the three products are just about the same."[4]

It is also a well known fact that simple or refined carbohydrates cause cavities. A recent study of cariogenicity (tooth decay), involving the analysis of eight honey samples, revealed that sucrose in the honey ranged from 0% to 3.0%, glucose from 33.1% to 41.5%, fructose from 42.8% to 50.7% and total sugar from 78.7% to 85.2%. When four groups of rats were fed either a sugar-free control diet, a diet with 18% sucrose, 18% honey or 18% mixed sugars (sucrose, glucose and fructose as found in honey) the controls exhibited significantly less caries in first and second molars than the other three groups. There were no significant differences among the three sugar groups in either the frequency or extent of cavities.[5] Honey, then, is at least as cavity producing as sucrose, and when eaten in combination with starchy foods is highly cariogenic.

RED MEATS

This may be one of the most difficult foods for many people to avoid since we in the Western world are heavy meat eaters. According to the U.S. Department of Agriculture, beef consumption in the United States was 55 pounds per person in 1940 and rose to 117 pounds per person by 1974. Our relative affluence and emphasis on protein has had much to do with our meat-eating habit.

What's wrong with red meat and why should it be avoided? Let's take a closer look at the various problems involved in the habitual consumption of beef, veal, pork, and lamb.

Red Meat and Heart Disease: Coronary artery disease is the leading cause of death in this country. According to the now well-known Framingham Study, in Framingham, Massachusetts which involved 5,200 cases, patients who have high serum cholesterol and triglycerides (fats in the blood), increase the risk of developing heart disease and other degenerative disorders.[6] Red meat, needless to say, is very high in fat. A steak, for example, yields about 75% of its total calories in fat.

A study of California Adventists showed that male Seventh-Day Adventists suffered their first heart attack a full decade later than most Americans, and the incidence of heart disease was only 60% of the average California male population.[7] The significance of this data is that most Seventh-Day Adventists are vegetarians.

Waste Products: Red meat contains waste products among which urea and uric acid are very prominent. High uric acid levels (hyperuricemia) have a tendency to increase the incidence of gout, or gouty arthritis.

Antibiotics and Hormones: In the past, cattle grazed freely in pastures, but today livestock raisers keep the majority penned up in a feedlot for several months before slaughtering time. The growers feed the animals natural and synthetic foods, including hormones, tranquilizers, and antibiotics such as tetracycline, streptomycin, dihydrostreptomycin, sulfonamides, and penicillin. DES (dithylstilbesterol) the synthetic estrogenic hormone used to fatten cattle has been isolated as a carcinogen (cancer producing).

Leukemia: Dr. Gordon H. Theilen, University of California School of Veterinary Medicine said, ''We have found that leukemia (an increase in the number of abnormal white blood cells) in cattle is being seen more frequently on certain farms. It's easy for meat inspectors to identify the terminal clinical form, but the microscopic leukemic stage will be missed every time if there is no gross enlargement, since blood studies are not conducted before slaughter.''[8]

Friendly Intestinal Bacteria: Nathan Pritikin points out that a diet emphasizing large amounts of animal products changes the intestinal flora (bacteria), destroying some friendly intestinal bacteria in the process.

Contamination: The U.S. Department of Agriculture establishes sanitation standards for 4,000 interstate meat and poultry plants. But inspectors condemn only about one–half of one percent of the meat brought to the plants. The government checked up on its meat inspection system in June, 1970, and found that thirty of the forty interstate meat plants visited by representatives of the U.S. General Accounting Office were violating sanitation standards.

In these plants, the GAO found cow or pig carcasses contaminated with cockroaches, flies, rodents, livestock stomach contents, mouse droppings, rust or moisture. This report was particularly alarming because the forty plants slaughter about 8% of all cattle and swine sold on the market, and included plants owned by such prestigious firms as Swift & Co., Wilson & Company, Inc., John Morrell & Co., Armour & Co., Carnation Co., Cudahy Co., and Stark, Wetzel & Co., Inc.[9]

Stoy Proctor, author of the book *Unmeat, a Case for Vegetarianism*, points out: ''It is common practice among livestock raisers to send sick animals to market before they become unsalable corpses. Even when inspectors do examine the meat, the processing plant often cuts off and discards the diseased area, then prepares the rest of the costly carcass for human consumption. Some have tried to argue that this practice is no different from cutting a bad spot out of an apple, but anyone familiar with physiology will recognize the difference. Animals have no isolated areas, for the blood and lymph move freely throughout the entire body.''[10]

One of the most common diseases transmitted from animals to human beings as a result of eating meat is brucellosis (undulant fever). The disease is contracted primarily by ingesting unpasteurized milk and through contact with infected cattle, pigs, and goats.

Another common condition is trichinosis, acquired by consuming raw or insufficiently cooked pork infected with tiny worms.

In 1972, the Department of Agriculture reported finding more than fifty different diseases in animals that were sent to the butcher's block.[11] All of this is reason enough to avoid meat. As someone once said, ''It's nice to sit down to a meal and not have to worry about what it died from.''

EXCESS PROTEIN

Just how much protein do we actually need in our diet? Research shows that we need much less than we think. The report published by the 1980 National Research Council of Food and Nutrition, recommends the following daily intake of protein:

Fig 4–3

	Age (years)	Protein (grams)
Children	1–3	23
	4–6	30
	7–10	34

	Age (years)	Protein (grams)
Males	11–14	45
	15–18	56
	19–22	56
	23–50	56
	51 +	56
Females	11–14	46
	15–18	46
	19–22	44
	23–50	44
	51 +	44
Pregnant	—	30 additional
Lactating	—	20 additional

Even though the Sensible Diet recommends limiting consumption of red meats, fish, and poultry, all of which are high in protein, it is still a relatively simple matter to meet your protein requirements. After determining what your protein requirements are, the next step is to find out whether you are meeting them. The accompanying list of foods and their protein values will assist you in making this determination.

As you can see, it's relatively simple to meet your protein requirements. However, sometimes it's very difficult to convince people of this because they've been so conditioned to think that to be healthy one must eat a great deal of protein. Conditions where increased consumption of protein might be justified are kwashiorkor (protein deficiency), infectious hepatitis, ulcerative colitis, prolonged diarrhea, and anemia.[12]

If you are reasonably healthy, eating more than the recommended amounts of protein will not make you any healthier

FIG. 4–4

PROTEIN VALUES OF COMMON FOODS

	Amount	Protein (grams)
DAIRY PRODUCTS		
Milk (non-fat)	1 cup	9
Milk (low-fat)	1 cup	10
Cottage cheese (low-fat)	1 cup	31
Mozzarella cheese (made from part skim milk)	1 ounce	8
Swiss cheese	1 ounce	8
Yogurt (low-fat)	1 cup	8
Eggs	1 egg	6
VEGETABLES, NUTS, BEANS, AND PEAS		
Almonds (shelled)	1 cup	26
Beans (red kidney)	1 cup	15
Peas (split/dry)	1 cup	20
Peas (green)	1 cup	9
Sunflower seeds	1 cup	24
Broccoli	1 stalk	6
Spinach (cooked)	1 cup	5
Apricots (dried)	1 cup	8
Tomato	1 medium	2

	Amount	Protein (grams)
GRAIN PRODUCTS		
Rye bread	1 slice	2
Barley (uncooked)	1 cup	16
Oatmeal or rolled oats	1 cup	5
Rice (white/cooked)	1 cup	4
MEAT, POULTRY, AND FISH		
Chicken (broiled)	1/2 breast	20
Steak (sirloin/broiled)	3 ounces	20
Tuna	3 ounces	24
Swordfish (broiled)	3 ounces	23

or stronger and may even cause problems. High protein intake has been implicated in such diverse disorders as kidney failure, gout, osteoporosis, breast cancer, bowel cancer, cancer of the pancreas, liver cirrhosis, obesity, reduced life expectancy, atherosclerosis, and lack of endurance.[13]

Another question I'm asked quite frequently is: Are large amounts of protein essential to athletes in training?

Many of the professional athletes whom I counsel are under the impression that they require large amounts of protein. Many feel that strenuous or vigorous physical activity results in protein loss because of the "wear and tear" on muscles. However, if this assumption were true, the body, in breaking down protein, which consists of carbon, hydrogen, oxygen, and nitrogen, would excrete nitrogen in the form of urea. Ellington Darden, of the Food and Nutrition Department, Florida State University, points out that numerous experiments on nitrogen balance indicate that the amount of nitrogen the body secretes after vigorous exercise is not significantly higher than the amounts excreted when the body has been resting. He adds that cross-country skiers, for example, who raced from twenty-two to fifty-three miles in one day excreted no more nitrogen following this workout than following sleep or rest.[14]

Another interesting study was done by Per-Olof Astrand, M.D., who conducted experiments to determine the best diet for athletes. He gave nine male subjects a mixed diet of protein, fat, and carbohydrate, and found that they could pedal a bicycle one hour and fifty-four minutes before exhaustion. Then, after three days on a diet high in fat and protein (meat, eggs, and milk), the subjects again exercised on the bicycles. This time they pedaled an average of only fifty-seven minutes before becoming exhausted.

Next, the nine participants followed a high complex-carbohydrate diet, such as the Sensible Diet, for three days before again exercising on the stationary bicycles. The men were then able to pedal an average of two hours and forty-seven minutes—

FIG. 4–5

ENDURANCE COMPARISONS FOR THREE BASIC DIETS

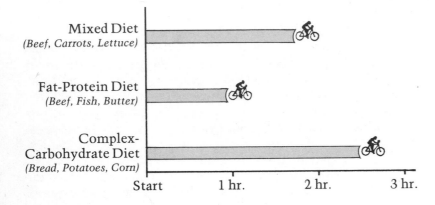

Mixed Diet
(Beef, Carrots, Lettuce)

Fat-Protein Diet
(Beef, Fish, Butter)

Complex-
Carbohydrate Diet
(Bread, Potatoes, Corn)

Start   1 hr.   2 hr.   3 hr.

almost two hours longer than when they were on the meat and dairy products diet. Some of the men on the complex-carbohydrate diet managed to continue for as long as four hours.[15]

It becomes clear on the basis of all of these facts that if a large part of your diet is comprised of animal protein, it would be in your best interests to decrease your protein intake. A heavy protein consumption is not essential, and red meats are not necessary to make you feel strong. If you still feel the need to sit down to a big steak once in a while, then go ahead, but consider that to be your splurge for the week.

SALT

Excessive salt can cause fluid retention in some people and may also increase blood pressure. Normal individuals promptly excrete excess sodium, no matter how high their dietary intake. However, in certain conditions, sodium cannot be eliminated. Additional water will then be held in the body to keep the sodium concentration of the fluid at a constant level. As a result, swelling of the tissues (edema) occurs.

The average American consumes approximately eight grams of salt per day which is far too much. The daily recommended intake has not been established; however, it appears that about one gram per day is all that's necessary unless a great deal of salt is lost through perspiration.

Are salt tablets necessary? Generally speaking, no. The old idea that salt tablets are necessary when exercising in hot weather no longer holds true. If you're going to be exercising in an area or environment where you are likely to be perspiring excessively, you might consider an electrolyte drink. Otherwise, drink plenty of water. Remember, there's salt in just about everything—including water, unless of course it's distilled.

Too much salt can be detrimental, particularly if you have heart disease, edema (fluid retention), hypertension, or are trying to lose weight. However, salt is also an essential mineral which is necessary for water balance, acid-base balance, nerve irritability, muscle contraction, and osmotic pressure. So, I am not recommending the elimination of salt altogether. That would be quite difficult in any case since salt is present in most foods we eat. What I am recommending is that you reduce your salt intake as much as possible by slowly re-acclimating your taste buds. You can start by reducing or eliminating the salt you normally add to food when cooking or at the table. At the same time, you can reduce your intake of foods that contain large amounts of sodium. (See Fig. 4–6.)

FIG. 4-6

FOODS HIGH IN SALT (SODIUM)

Meat, Meat Flavorings, and Fish

Anchovies
Bacon
Bacon fat
Canned meats
Caviar
Corned beef
Dried cod
Frankfurters
Ham
Herring

Luncheon meats
Meat extracts
Meat sauces
Meat tenderizers
Salted and smoked fish
Salted and smoked meats
Sardines
Sausages
Tuna (canned in oil)

Appetizers, Sauces, and Seasonings

Cheeses
Celery salt
Chili sauce
Garlic salt
Ketchup
Mustard
Olives
Onion salt
Pickles
Potato chips

Pretzels
Regular bouillon cubes
Relishes
Salted nuts
Salted popcorn
Sauerkraut
Soy sauce
Table salt
Worcestershire sauce

FOODS MODERATELY HIGH IN SALT (SODIUM)

Breads and Cereals

Breads
Corn flakes
Crackers

Rolls
Waffles

Vegetables

Canned vegetables
Canned vegetable juices
Celery

Dairy Products

Cheese
Salted butter
Salted margarine

Meat and Fish

Clams
Crabs
Kidneys
Lobsters
Oysters
Scallops
Shrimp

Other

Baking powder
Beverage mixes
Molasses
Salad dressings
Water
   (distilled water has *no* sodium)

TABLE SALTS

Plain salt: 100% sodium chloride
Iodized Salt: 100% sodium chloride with iodine added
Light Salt: 50% sodium chloride and 50% potassium chloride
Salt Substitute: 100% potassium chloride. Large amounts of
   potassium chloride may cause irregular heart beats. Do not
   use without consulting your doctor.

SATURATED FATS

Avoid saturated fats as much as possible. The average American eats a diet that contains about 45% fat. Saturated fats are generally derived from animal sources and are normally solid or firm at room temperature, whereas polyunsaturated fats are generally from a plant source, and are normally liquid or soft at room temperature. The exceptions are coconut oil, palm kernel oil and chocolate fat (cocoa butter), all of which are saturated fats derived from plant material.

Eliminate rich salad dressings such as Roquefort and blue cheese. Use either lemon juice, apple cider vinegar, or herb dressings.

Also, don't be fooled by foods prepared with hydrogenated vegetable oils. Once an unsaturated fat is hydrogenated, i.e., artificially hardened, it becomes a saturated fat.

Saturated fats, when taken in excess, can not only elevate triglycerides, but may also elevate the amount of cholesterol normally found in the blood. Elevated cholesterol levels have been linked to atherosclerotic lesions (fatty deposits) that sometimes build up in the arteries, and restrict the flow of blood to the heart. It's this type of blockage in the arteries that may result in a heart attack or a stroke.

Recent evidence has shown that polyunsaturated fats are not necessarily safer than saturated fats. Dr. Meyer Friedman and his associates in San Francisco demonstrated that unsaturated fats in the diet produced just as much fat blockage in the capillaries as ordinary animal fat and often stayed in the bloodstream longer than saturated fats. One of Dr. Friedman's studies, documented in the *Journal of the American Medical Association*, involved forty firemen from San Francisco. To determine blockages, photographs were taken of the small blood vessels in the subjects' eyes. Before eating or drinking, the vessels were wide open—there were no blockages. Dr. Friedman then gave each of the subjects a glass of heavy cream. Five hours after the cream drink, approximately twenty-five blockages were found in the eyes of these subjects. Later, after the blood vessels had cleared, the subjects were given safflower oil, a polyunsaturated fat. Five hours after the oil drink, there were just as many blockages of the same severity as after the cream drink. Dr. Friedman's conclusion was that substituting polyunsaturated fats for saturated fats is not the solution to the problem of blood vessel blockage, since both block the small blood vessels. He urged the reduction of *all* fats.[16]

In another study, Dr. Marvin Bierenbaum and his associates in New Jersey performed a similar experiment with 200 men who had already had heart attacks. The results showed that unsaturated fats are no better at alleviating the risks of subsequent heart attacks than are saturated fats.[17]

FRIED FOODS

Avoid fried foods. Frying foods not only increases caloric content, but also increases fat content. Recommendations: steam, broil, or bake.

SOFT DRINKS *(Sweetened/Carbonated)*

In addition to containing too much sugar, empty calories, artificial colorings, and in some instances corrosive agents, soft drinks contain too much phosphorus. There is a good possibility that too much phosphorus may upset the calcium-phosphorus balance, and possibly lead to osteoporosis (porous and fragile bones). Some soft drinks have more phosphorus than others and some also contain caffeine.

ALCOHOLIC BEVERAGES

Hard liquor is not recommended; however, an occasional glass of beer or wine is acceptable.

COFFEE AND TEA

Herb teas without caffeine are an exception. An occasional cup of decaffeinated coffee is permissible. The primary ingredient of concern in coffee and tea is caffeine. Caffeine is not recommended for the following reasons:

1. There is evidence that caffeine ingested daily over a long period of time increases an individual's susceptibility to coronary heart disease by increasing free fatty acids through central nervous system stimulation.[18]

2. Caffeine increases gastric secretions which may eventually induce ulcers.[19]

3. Caffeine may cause complications in delivery.[20]

4. Caffeine may cause miscarriages or birth defects and should be avoided by pregnant women, according to the Center for Science in the Public Interest in Washington, D.C.

5. There is also speculation that caffeine-containing substances deplete some of the B vitamins, but the evidence to support this is inconclusive.

Which contains more caffeine—coffee or tea? Ounce per ounce, dry tea has more caffeine than dry coffee. However, we have to keep in mind that it takes more dry ingredient to make a cup of coffee than it does to make a cup of tea. So if we're measuring both substances in liquid form, one cup of coffee would contain more. However, if the measurements are made in dry form, ounce per ounce, tea contains more caffeine.

CANNED AND PRESERVED FOODS

Avoid foods that have been canned or preserved. Use discretion with frozen foods. Frozen TV dinners, for example, are definitely to be avoided.

FOODS HIGH IN CHOLESTEROL

There have been innumerable investigations and epidemiological studies performed linking elevated cholesterol levels with coronary artery disease. The recommendation for decrease in the consumption of foods that are high in cholesterol is based on the results of these investigations.

Foods that have the highest cholesterol content are organ meats (liver, brains, kidneys), egg yolks, dairy products, and shellfish. Use the chart on Cholesterol Content (Fig. 4–7) to determine the cholesterol levels of many common foods. The recommended goal is to keep your cholesterol below 160 mg. Most laboratories consider 150 to 300 mg. to be normal. The lower your cholesterol level, the better. If you don't know what your cholesterol level is, request a blood test, and ask for the results.

Cholesterol is a steroid used by the body in small amounts in the manufacture of hormones. It is probably the most pertinent blood value to monitor. Artery closure and heart disease are rarely found in populations in which the average cholesterol remains under 160 mg. throughout adult life. Dr. Cleaves Bennett, Medical Director of the Longevity Center in Santa Monica, California, states that, "In our country, where the average cholesterol level of adults is 240 mg., almost all patients who die of heart disease have cholesterol levels in the U.S. normal range."[21]

The following is a case history which documents the importance of a low cholesterol diet:

Most people remember Dr. Philip Blaiberg, the South African dentist, at one time the longest surviving heart transplant patient. He died nineteen months after his heart transplant, not of tissue rejection, as people thought at first, but of a heart attack. The doctor who examined Blaiberg's heart after he died found the heart's arteries choked with atherosclerosis. This same doctor had examined the new heart before the transplant and knew that the arteries were as clean as a baby's at that time.

During the entire nineteen months with his new heart, Dr. Blaiberg maintained a high level of blood cholesterol. It started out at 315 and never dropped below 300. The kind of food that Blaiberg needed to drop his cholesterol level to a low value was never provided him. The diet that destroyed his first heart did just as effective a job destroying his second heart.[22]

Findings established by the Framingham Study have confirmed the correlation between elevated cholesterol levels and atherosclerosis.

Ansel Keys's lengthy seven-country study involving 13,000 men from around the world also confirmed the relationship between elevated cholesterol levels and atherosclerosis.[23]

Serum cholesterol has proven remarkably successful as an indicator of coronary heart disease risk as confirmed by motion picture angiography.[24] C.C. Welch utilized this technique to study 723 men under forty, all of whom underwent cinecoronary angiography because of chest pain. Of the patients studied, 49% were found to have an average of two main branches of the coronary arteries significantly narrowed (more than 50% closure). The percent of closure was found to be directly related to serum cholesterol levels.[25]

There is also a very common misconception regarding cholesterol. Dietary cholesterol is *not* our sole source of cholesterol. The body produces about 75% of our serum cholesterol. This does not mean, however, that the restriction of dietary cholesterol is not important, but only that the body itself already produces a large proportion of this substance.

FIG. 4–7

CHOLESTEROL CONTENT

Approximate Amounts of Cholesterol in Milligrams Per 100 Gram (3½ Oz.) Portions of Foods

Beef		Fish	
Rump roast	58	Trout	57
Round steak	68	Tuna	51
Chuck roast	55	Salmon	55
Veal	71	Halibut	33
Pork		Haddock	64
Chops	55	Codfish	46
Tenderloin	57	Mackerel	80
Ham	42	Herring	75
Lamb		Perch	63
Chops	66	Pike	71
Mutton	77	**Shellfish**	
Turkey		Shrimp	161
Light	61	Crab	99
Dark	96	Lobster	83
Chicken		Oysters	161
Light	54	Scallops	166
Dark	76	Clams	118
Kidney	300	**Milk**	
Liver, beef	320	Whole	14
Brains, calf	1810	Fortified skim	
Sweetbreads	280	(1% butterfat)	5
Beef tallow	56	Skim	< 1
Lard	65	Buttermilk	6

Cheeses		Butter	249
Limburger	92	**Cream**	
Roquefort	73	Thick	140
Cream	140	Thin	40
American Process	87	**Egg yolks**	1370
Cheddar	98	(1 egg yolk)	240
Bleu	157		
Mozzarella (part skim)	61		
Swiss	91		
Gouda	33		
Hoop	1		
Parmesan	74		
American	92		

Amounts of Cholesterol in Milligrams Per Serving of Food

1 cup fortified skim milk (less than 1% buttermilk fat)	12	1 egg yolk	240
		1 tsp. butter	10
		1 Tbsp. mayonnaise	15
1 cup fortified skim milk (less than 0.5% butterfat)	6	1 Tbsp. thick cream	18
		Margarine, vegetable	0
		Peanut butter	0
1 cup skim milk	1	Fruits	0
½ cup sherbert	3	Vegetables	0
1 cup whole milk	35	Egg whites	0
½ cup ice cream	30	Cereals	0
½ cup ice milk	17	Vegetable oils	0

From ''Low Cholesterol Diet Manual,'' Department of Internal Medicine, University of Iowa.

The Pure Water Controversy

Drink plenty of fresh spring or well water. Why only fresh spring or well water? In the words of Kant, ''It is often necessary to make a decision on the basis of knowledge sufficient for action, but insufficient to satisfy the intellect.'' Unfortunately there is still much scientific uncertainty surrounding the carcinogen question. I have to admit, even as a health professional, I get tired of hearing that this may cause cancer or that may cause cancer. After a while, you begin to feel that everything you touch, breathe, and eat is cancer-causing. But like it or not, it's a reality.

The controversy over the safety of drinking water centers around three classes of chemicals: fluoride, polychlorinated biphenyls (PCBs) and trihalomethanes (THMs).

Let's start with fluoride, which has long been the object of controversy. To fluoridate, or not to fluoridate—that is the question. Fluoridated water, according to Dr. John Yiamouyiannis of the National Health Federation, has been linked to cancer.[26] Dr. Dean Burk, former head of the National Cancer Institute's cytochemistry section, has also had similar findings.[27]

Most dental and public health authorities seem to disagree. They claim that there is insufficient evidence to link cancer to the fluoride in our water supplies. Proponents of fluoride also claim that it reduces the incidence of dental caries. Albert Burgstahler, Ph.D., Department of Chemistry, University of Kansas, in a presentation to the House of Representatives on October 12, 1977, stated that, ''Despite whatever reduction in tooth decay can be achieved by fluoridation, there is a steadily growing amount of solid evidence showing that fluoride in drinking water at the officially recommended concentration of 0.7 to 1.2 ppm (parts per million) causes serious harmful effects in its users.''[28]

Opponents also argue that altering the community water supply is ''unnatural'' and deprives its consumers of their freedom of choice. Those who want fluoride can get it by way of drops, tablets, toothpaste, or dental treatments; leaving those who do not want it free to choose. Others fear accidental overdoses. Fluorine is a highly volatile chemical and is deadly in excess.[29]

The other two classes of chemicals are PCBs and THMs. Both have been found in our drinking water, and both have been shown to be cancer producing. Not only are these chemicals fed into the water supply by industry, but they are also produced by standard water treatment procedures!

WHAT ABOUT BOTTLED WATER?

Most bottled waters are fine. There are, however, a few things to look for. First, read the labels to see exactly what the water does or doesn't contain. Switching from tap to bottled water may not necessarily guarantee better water quality. In fact, you might in some cases be paying higher prices for bottles of the very tap water you're trying to avoid.

Second, find out where the water came from. When the Environmental Protective Agency surveyed fifty water bottlers a few years ago about the source of their water, their responses were as follows:

21 said it came from tap water.

13 got their water from wells.

10 were supplied by springs.

4 used imported water.

2 combined waters from more than one source.

It's not surprising that many bottlers don't indicate the source of their waters on their labels.

Is bottled water chlorinated? With just a few exceptions, bottled water is chlorinated, but then the chlorine is removed before it's bottled.

WELL WATER

Well water is also recommended, as long as it meets the standards set up by the Environmental Protection Agency. (Although the EPA does not require bottling companies to indicate its approval on the container, the company must receive this approval in order to be licensed.)

DISTILLED WATER

The use of distilled water is optional. It is produced by heating water into vapor, then allowing it to condense into liquid again —pretty much the way rain is made. Distillation removes most solids, minerals, and trace elements. Therefore, if you decide to buy distilled water, keep in mind that the mineral levels are either negligible, or in very small quantities. This is one reason why distilled water is often recommended for low sodium diets.

Is distilled water chlorinated? No, it's not. Since distilled water is never contaminated, chlorination isn't necessary.

WHAT ABOUT MINERAL WATER?

Mineral water, such as Perrier, is actually considered to be carbonated water, i.e., it mixes with underground gases before it reaches the earth's surface. Perrier with a wedge of lime is fine once in a while. It's generally agreed that you should not drink *only* carbonated water. It is not meant to be a substitute for tap or bottled water. Most carbonated mineral waters, such as San Pellegrino, Vichy Celestins, Appolinaris, Badoit, and Saratoga Vichy, are not only unavailable to most consumers, but are too expensive as well.

PURIFIED WATER

Purified water is any water that has had its impurities removed. One process according to Paul Williams, Quality Control Manager for Arrowhead Waters in Los Angeles, is reverse osmosis, followed by deionization (RO-DI). Reverse osmosis is a process that employs a filtering unit with a semi-permeable membrane which allows pure water molecules to pass through it while rejecting up to 98% of dissolved salts, mercury, chlorine, nitrates and sulfates. In addition, it successfully removes DDT, detergents, algae, harmful bacteria and chemical wastes, as well as all undissolved particles.

If you've heard that purified water harms the body by leaching minerals from it, don't believe it. There's no basis for this statement, nor any scientific evidence to support it.

Considering all the problems associated with other drinking waters, the preferred choices come down to fresh spring bottled water or an EPA approved well water. If you are not able to purchase bottled water for whatever reasons, then let tap water be your second choice.

Ingredients and Additives

A nutritionally oriented person should be aware that labels don't always tell the full story. There is no legal requirement that the actual amounts of various ingredients in food products be given. They are required to be listed however, in decreasing order of quantity. That is, if there is more sugar than grain contained in a box of cereal, the sugar must be listed first.

Many food companies will often combine the grains and split the sugar content, by listing each type separately. That way sugar seldom appears as the first ingredient. They will list table sugar, brown sugar, dextrose, molasses, and honey separately, knowing full well that there is not a great deal of difference in the way our bodies receive them.

The fact is that brown sugar, which customarily gets its color from the addition of caramel color, is basically the same as table sugar. Brown sugar is white sugar with some of the molasses put back. It has some trace elements, true, but the carbohydrate content is virtually the same as white sugar.

There are over 2,700 food additives being used in foods, as of this writing. Some of these additives are harmful and some ar not. (See Fig. 4-9 to determine which food additives are safe.) As a general rule, try to avoid foods with long lists of unpronounceable ingredients. Also keep in mind that the wider the variety of foods that you eat, the greater will be the variety of different chemical substances consumed, thus reducing the chance that any one chemical will reach a hazardous level.[30] This is assuming, of course, that you do not try to subsist on a diet of hot dogs, soft drinks, potato chips and maraschino cherries.

Recently, the food additives that have received considerable attention are artificial colorings, artificial flavorings, nitrates and nitrites. Artificial colorings and flavorings have been in the limelight primarily as a result of the studies advanced by Dr. Ben Feingold on the relationship of these substances to hyperactivity in children. Nitrates and nitrites have been of concern because of their possible link to cancer.

FIG. 4-8

AVERAGE U.S. CONSUMPTION OF NITRITE PER PERSON PER DAY

Source	Nitrite (mg)
Vegetables	198
Cured meat	2,380
Saliva	8,620

Nitrates and nitrites can combine with amines in the stomach to form nitrosamines, which are cancer-causing substances. However, what most people don't know is that nitrites occur naturally in some vegetables as well as in saliva. The amount of nitrites occuring naturally in the body is actually much higher than the average daily consumption of nitrite in bacon, ham and hot dogs.[31] (See Fig. 4–8.) The problem, then, is not with the nitrates (which are converted to nitrites during the meat-curing process) or the nitrites themselves, but with the overconsumption of these substances.

The following information on chemicals and additives are broken down into three categories: Those which are safe, those which are to be used with caution, and those which should be avoided.

* *Chemical Cuisine* reprinted with permission of The Center for Science in the Public Interest. Washington, D.C. © 1978, CSPI.

FIG. 4–9

Chemical Cuisine*

SAFE

The following additives appear to be safe:

ALGINATE, PROPYLENE GLYCOL ALGINATE

FUNCTION: Thickening agents; foam stabilizer.
USED IN: *Ice cream, cheese, candy, yogurt.*

Alginate, an apparently safe derivative of seaweed (kelp) maintains the desired texture in dairy products, canned frosting, and other factory-made foods. **Propylene glycol alginate,** a chemically-modified algin, thickens acidic foods (soda pop, salad dressing) and stabilizes the foam in beer.

ALPHA TOCOPHEROL (Vitamin E)

FUNCTION: Antioxidant, nutrient.
USED IN: *Vegetable oil.*

Vitamin E is abundant in whole wheat, rice germ, and vegetable oils. It is destroyed by the refining and bleaching of flour. Vitamin E prevents oils from going rancid.

ASCORBIC ACID (Vitamin C),

FUNCTION: **ERYTHORBIC ACID** Antioxidant, nutrient, color stabilizer.
USED IN: *Oily foods, cereals, soft drinks, cured meats.*

Ascorbic acid helps maintain the red color of cured meat and prevents the formation of nitrosamines (see sodium nitrate). It helps prevent loss of color and flavor by reacting with unwanted oxygen. It is used as a nutrient additive in drinks and breakfast cereals. **Sodium ascorbate** is a more soluble form of ascorbic acid. **Erythorbic acid** (sodium erythorbate) serves the same functions as ascorbic acid, but has no value as a vitamin.

BETA CAROTENE

FUNCTION: Coloring; nutrient.
USED IN: *Margarine, shortening, non-dairy whiteners, butter.*

Used as an artificial coloring and a nutrient supplement. The body converts it to Vitamin A, which is part of the light-detection mechanism of the eye.

CALCIUM (or SODIUM) PROPIONATE

FUNCTION: Preservative.
USED IN: *Bread, rolls, pies, cakes.*

Calcium propionate prevents mold growth on bread and rolls. The calcium is a beneficial mineral; the propionate is safe. **Sodium propionate** is used in pies and cakes, because calcium alters the action of chemical leavening agents.

CALCIUM (or SODIUM) STEAROYL LACTYLATE

FUNCTION: Dough conditioner, whipping agent.
USED IN: *Bread dough, cake fillings, artificial whipped cream, processed egg whites.*

These additives strengthen bread dough so it can be used in bread-making machinery and lead to more uniform grain and greater volume. They act as whipping agents in dried, liquid, or frozen egg whites and artificial whipped cream. **Sodium stearoyl fumarate** serves the same function.

CARRAGEENAN

FUNCTION: Thickening and stabilizing agent.
USED IN: *Ice cream, jelly, chocolate milk, infant formula.*

Obtained from "Irish Moss" seaweed, it is used as a thickening agent and to stabilize oil-water mixtures.

CASEIN, SODIUM CASEINATE

FUNCTION: Thickening and whitening agent.
USED IN: *Ice cream, ice milk, sherbet, coffee creamers.*

Casein, the principal protein in milk, is a nutritious protein containing adequate amounts of all the essential amino acids.

CITRIC ACID, SODIUM CITRATE

FUNCTION: Acid, flavoring, chelating agent.
USED IN: *Ice cream, sherbet, fruit drink, candy, carbonated beverages, instant potatoes.*

Citric acid is versatile, widely used, cheap, and safe. It is an important metabolite in virtually all living organisms; especially abundant in citrus fruits and berries. It is used as a strong acid, a tart flavoring, and an antioxidant. **Sodium citrate,** also safe, is a buffer that controls the acidity of gelatin deserts, jam, ice cream, candy, and other foods.

EDTA

FUNCTION: Chelating agent.
USED IN: *Salad dressing, margarine, sandwich spreads, mayonnaise, processed fruits and vegetables, canned shellfish, soft drinks.*

Modern food manufacturing technology, which involves metal rollers, blenders, and containers, results in trace amounts of metal contamination in food. **EDTA** (ethylene-diamine tetraacetic acid) traps metal impurities, which would otherwise promote rancidity and the breakdown of artificial colors.

FERROUS GLUCONATE

FUNCTION: Coloring, nutrient.
USED IN: *Black olives.*

Used by the olive industry to generate a uniform jet-black color and in pills as a source of iron. Safe.

FUMARIC ACID

FUNCTION: Tartness agent.
USED IN: *Powdered drinks, pudding, pie fillings, gelatin desserts.*

A solid at room temperature, inexpensive, highly acidic, it is the ideal source of tartness and acidity in dry food products. However, it dissolves slowly in cold water, a drawback cured by adding **Dioctyl sodium sulfosuccinate (DSS),** a poorly tested, detergent-like additive.

GELATIN

FUNCTION: Thickening and gelling agent.
USED IN: *Powdered dessert mix, yogurt, ice cream, cheese spreads, beverages.*

Gelatin is a protein obtained from animal bones, hoof, and other parts. It has little nutritional value, because it contains little or none of several amino acids.

GLYCERIN (GLYCEROL)

FUNCTION: Maintains water content.
USED IN: *Marshmallow, candy, fudge, baked goods.*

Glycerin forms the backbone of fat and oil molecules and is quite safe. The body uses it as a source of energy or as a starting material in making more complex molecules.

HYDROLYZED VEGETABLE PROTEIN (HVP)

FUNCTION: Flavor enhancer.
USED IN: *Instant soups, frankfurters, sauce mixes, beef stew.*

HVP consists of vegetable (usually soybean) protein that has been chemically broken down to the amino acids of which it is composed. HVP is used to bring out the natural flavor of food (and, perhaps, to use less real food).

LACTIC ACID

FUNCTION: Acidity regulator.
USED IN: *Spanish olives, cheese, frozen desserts, carbonated beverage.*

This safe acid occurs in almost all living organisms. It inhibits spoilage in Spanish-type olives, balances the acidity in cheese-making, and adds tartness to frozen desserts, carbonated fruit-flavored drinks and other foods.

LACTOSE

FUNCTION: Sweetener.
USED IN: *Whipped topping mix, breakfast pastry.*

Lactose, a carbohydrate found only in milk, is nature's way of delivering calories to infant mammals.

One-sixth as sweet as table sugar, it is added to food as a slightly sweet source of carbohydrate. Milk turns sour when bacteria converts lactose to lactic acid.

LECITHIN

FUNCTION: Emulsifier, antioxidant.
USED IN: *Baked goods, margarine, chocolate, ice cream.*

A common constituent of animal and plant tissues, it is a source of the nutrient choline. It keeps oil and water from separating out, retards rancidity, reduces spattering in a frying pan and leads to fluffier cakes. Major sources are egg yolk and soybeans.

MANNITOL

FUNCTION: Sweetener, other uses.
USED IN: *Chewing gum, low-calorie foods.*

Not quite as sweet as sugar and poorly absorbed by the body, it contributes only half as many calories as sugar. Used as the "dust" on chewing gum, it prevents gum from absorbing moisture and becoming sticky. Safe.

MONO- and DIGLYCERIDES

FUNCTION: Emulsifiers.
USED IN: *Baked goods, margarine, candy, peanut butter.*

Makes bread softer and prevents staling, improves the stability of margarine, makes caramels less sticky, and prevents the oil in peanut butter from separating out. **Mono- and diglycerides** are safe, though most foods they are used in are high in refined flour, sugar or fat.

POLYSORBATE 60

FUNCTION: Emulsifier.
USED IN: *Baked goods, frozen desserts, imitation dairy products.*

Polysorbate 60 is short for polyoxyethylene-(20)-sorbitan monostearate. It and its close relatives, Polysorbate 65 and 80, are synthetic, but appear to be safe. These chemicals work the same way as mono- and diglycerides, but smaller amounts are needed. They keep baked goods from going stale, keep dill oil dissolved in bottled dill pickles, help coffee whiteners dissolve in coffee, and prevent oil from separating out of artificial whipped cream.

SODIUM BENZOATE

USED IN: *Fruit juice, carbonated drinks, pickles, preserves.*

Manufacturers have used **sodium benzoate** for over 70 years to prevent the growth of micro-organisms in acidic foods.

SODIUM CARBOXYMETHYLCELLULOSE (CMC)

FUNCTION: Thickening and stabilizing agent; prevents sugar from crystallizing.
USED IN: *Ice cream, beer, pie fillings, icings, diet foods, candy.*

CMC is made by reacting cellulose with a derivative of acetic acid. Studies indicate it is safe.

SORBIC ACID, POTASSIUM SORBATE

FUNCTION: Prevents growth of mold and bacteria.
USED IN: *Cheese, syrup, jelly, cake, wine, dry fruits.*

Sorbic Acid occurs naturally in the berries of the mountain ash. **Sorbate** may be a safe replacement for sodium nitrite in bacon.

SORBITAN MONOSTEARATE

FUNCTION: Emulsifier.

USED IN: *Cakes, candy, frozen pudding, icing.*

Like mono- and diglycerides and poly-sorbates, this additive keeps oil and water mixed together. In chocolate candy, it prevents the discoloration that normally occurs when the candy is warmed up and then cooled down.

SORBITOL

FUNCTION: Sweetener, thickening agent, maintains moisture.

USED IN: *Dietetic drinks and foods; candy, shredded coconut, chewing gum.*

Sorbitol occurs naturally in fruits and berries and is a close relative of the sugars. It is half as sweet as sugar. It is used in non-cariogenic chewing gum because oral bacteria do not metabolize it well. Large amounts of sorbitol (2 oz for adults) have a laxative effect, but otherwise it is safe. Diabetics use sorbitol, because it is absorbed slowly and does not cause blood sugar to increase rapidly.

STARCH, MODIFIED STARCH

FUNCTION: Thickening agent.

USED IN: *Soup, gravy, baby foods.*

Starch, the major component of flour, potatoes, and corn, is used as a thickening agent. However, it does not dissolve in cold water. Chemists have solved this problem by reacting starch with various chemicals. These modified starches are added to some foods to improve their consistency and keep the solids suspended. Starch and modified starches make foods look thicker and richer than they really are.

VANILLIN, ETHYL VANILLIN

FUNCTION: Substitute for vanilla.

USED IN: *Ice cream, baked goods, beverages, chocolate, candy, gelatin desserts.*

Vanilla flavoring is derived from a bean, but **vanillin,** the major flavor component of vanilla, is cheaper to produce synthetically. A derivation, **ethyl vanillin,** comes closer to matching the taste of real vanilla. Vanillin is safe, ethyl vanillin needs to be better tested.

CAUTION

These additives may be unsafe, are poorly tested, or are used in foods we eat too much of:

ARTIFICIAL FLAVORING

FUNCTION: Flavoring.

USED IN: *Soda pop, candy, breakfast cereals, gelatin desserts; many others.*

Hundreds of chemicals are used to mimic natural flavors; many may be used in a single flavoring, such as for cherry soda pop. Most flavoring chemicals also occur in nature and are probably safe, but they may cause hyperactivity in some sensitive children. Artificial flavorings are used almost exclusively in junk foods; their use indicates that the real thing (usually fruit) has been left out.

BUTYLATED HYDROXYANISOLE (BHA)

FUNCTION: Antioxidant.

USED IN: *Cereals, chewing gum, potato chips, vegetable oil.*

BHA retards rancidity in fats, oils, and oil-containing foods. It appears to be safer than **BHT** (see additives to avoid), but needs to be better tested. This synthetic chemical can often be replaced by safer chemicals.

CORN SYRUP

FUNCTION: Sweetener, thickener.

USED IN: *Candy, toppings, syrups, snack foods, imitation dairy foods.*

Corn syrup is a sweet, thick liquid made by treating cornstarch with acids or enzymes. It may be dried and used as **corn syrup solids** in coffee whiteners, and other dry products. Corn syrup contains no nutritional value other than calcium, promotes tooth decay, and is used mainly in low-nutrition foods.

DEXTROSE (GLUCOSE, CORN SUGAR)

FUNCTION: Sweetener, coloring agent.

USED IN: *Bread, caramel, soda pop, cookies, many other foods.*

Dextrose is an important chemical in every living organism. A sugar, it is a source of sweetness in fruits and honey. Added to foods as a sweetener, it represents empty calories, and contributes to tooth decay. Dextrose turns brown when heated and contributes to the color of bread crust and toast.

GUMS: Guar, Locust Bean, Arabic, Furcelleran, Ghatti, Karaya, Tragacanth

FUNCTION: Thickening agents, stabilizers.

USED IN: *Beverages, ice cream, frozen pudding, salad dressing, dough, cottage cheese, candy, drink mixes.*

Gums derive from natural sources (bushes, trees or seaweed) and are poorly tested. They are used to thicken foods, prevent sugar crystals from forming in candy, stabilize beer foam (arabic), form a gel in pudding (furcelleran), encapsulate flavor oils in powdered drink mixes, or keep oil and water mixed together in salad dressings. Tragacanth, sometimes used in McDonald's "Big Macs" and many other foods, has caused occasional severe allergic reactions.

HEPTYL PARABEN

FUNCTION: Preservative
USED IN: *Beer*

Heptyl paraben—short for the heptyl ester of para-hydroxybenzoic acid—is used as a preservative in some beers. Studies suggest this chemical is safe, but it has not been tested in the presence of alcohol.

HYDROGENATED VEGETABLE OIL

FUNCTION: Source of oil or fat.
USED IN: *Margarine, many processed foods.*

Vegetable oil, usually a liquid, can be made into a semi-solid by treating with hydrogen. Unfortunately, hydrogenation converts much of the polyunsaturated oil to saturated fat. We eat too much oil and fat of all kinds, whether natural or hydrogenated. Additive needs better testing.

MONOSODIUM GLUTAMATE (MSG)

FUNCTION: Flavor enhancer.
USED IN: *Soup, seafood, cheese, sauces, stews; many others.*

This amino acid brings out the flavor of protein-containing foods. Large amounts of **MSG** fed to infant mice destroyed nerve cells in the brain. Public pressure forced baby food companies to stop using MSG. MSG causes ''Chinese Restaurant Syndrome'' (burning sensation in the back of the neck and forearms, tightness of the chest, headache) in some sensitive adults.

PHOSPHORIC ACID: PHOSPHATES

FUNCTION: Acidulant, chelating agent, buffer, emulsifier, nutrient, discoloration inhibitor.
USED IN: *Baked goods, cheese, powdered foods, cured meats, soda pop, breakfast cereals, dehydrated potatoes.*

Phosphoric acid acidifies and flavors cola beverages. Phosphate salts are used in hundreds of processed foods for many purposes. **Calcium** and **iron phosphates** act as mineral supplements. **Sodium aluminum phosphate** is a leavening agent. **Calcium and ammonium phosphates** serve as food for yeast in bread. **Sodium acid pyrophosphate** prevents discoloration in potatoes and sugar syrups. Phosphates are not toxic, but their widespread use has led to a dietary imbalance that may be causing osteoporosis.

SULFUR DIOXIDE, SODIUM BISULFITE

FUNCTION: Preservative, bleach.
USED IN: *Sliced fruit, wine, grape juice, dehydrated potatoes.*

Sulfur dioxide (a gas) and **sodium bisulfite** (a powder) prevent discoloration of dried apricots, apples and similar foods. They prevent bacterial growth in wine and other foods. These additives destroy vitamin B-1, but otherwise are safe.

AVOID

The additive is unsafe in the amounts consumed or is very poorly tested.

ARTIFICIAL COLORINGS

Most artificial colorings are synthetic chemicals that do not occur in nature. Though some are safer than others, colorings are not listcd by name on labels. Because colorings are used almost solely in foods of low nutritional value (candy, soda pop, gelatin desserts, etc.), you should simply avoid all artificially colored foods. In addition to problems mentioned below, there is evidence that colorings may cause hyperactivity in some sensitive children. The use of coloring usually indicates that fruit or other natural ingredient has not been used.

BLUE No. 1

FUNCTION: Artificial coloring.
USED IN: *Beverages, candy, baked goods.*

Very poorly tested; possible risk. Avoid.

BLUE No. 2

FUNCTION: Artificial coloring.
USED IN: *Pet food, beverages, candy.*

Very poorly tested; should be avoided.

CITRUS RED No. 2

FUNCTION: Artificial coloring.
USED IN: *Skin of some Florida oranges only.*

Studies indicate that this additive causes cancer. The dye does not seep through the orange skin into the pulp.

GREEN No. 3

FUNCTION: Artificial coloring.
USED IN: *Candy, beverages.*

Needs to be better tested; avoid.

ORANGE B

FUNCTION: Artificial coloring.
USED IN: *Hot dogs.*

Was used to color some hot dogs; the FDA had approved it in 1966, despite shamefully poor tests. In 1978 the producer stopped making it upon discovering that it contained a cancer-causing impurity.

RED No. 3

FUNCTION: Artificial coloring.
USED IN: *Cherries in fruit cocktail, candy, baked goods.*

This complex, synthetic dye may cause cancer.

RED No. 40

FUNCTION: Artificial coloring.
USED IN: *Soda pop, candy, gelatin desserts, pastry, pet food, sausage.*

The most widely used coloring promotes cancer in mice; should be avoided.

YELLOW No. 5

FUNCTION: Artificial coloring.
USED IN: *Gelatin dessert, candy, pet food, baked goods.*

The second most widely used coloring is poorly tested, with one test suggesting it might cause cancer. Some people are allergic to it.

YELLOW No. 6

FUNCTION: Artificial coloring.

USED IN: *Beverages, sausage, baked goods, candy, gelatin.*

Appears safe, but can cause occasional allergic reactions; used almost exclusively in junk foods.

BROMINATED VEGETABLE OIL (BVO)

FUNCTION: Emulsifier, clouding agent.

USED IN: *Soft drinks.*

BVO keeps flavor oils in suspension and gives a cloudy appearance to citrus-flavored soft drinks. The residues of **BVO** found in body fats are cause for concern. **BVO** should be banned; safer substitutes are available.

BUTYLATED HYDROXYTOLUENE (BHT)

FUNCTION: Antioxidant.

USED IN: *Cereals, chewing gum, potato chips, oils. etc.*

BHT is poorly tested, is found in body fat, and causes occasional allergic reactions. **BHT** is unnecessary in many of the foods in which it is used; safer alternatives are available.

CAFFEINE

FUNCTION: Stimulant

USED IN: *Coffee, tea, cocoa (natural); soft drinks (additive).*

Caffeine may cause birth defects and should be avoided by pregnant women. It also keeps many people from sleeping.

INVERT SUGAR

FUNCTION: Sweetener.

USED IN: *Candy, soft drinks, many other foods.*

Invert sugar, a 50-50 mixture of two sugars, dextrose and fructose, is sweeter and more soluble than sucrose (table sugar). Invert sugar forms when sucrose is split in two by an enzyme or acid. It represents "empty calories," contributes to tooth decay, and should be avoided.

PROPYL GALLATE

FUNCTION: Antioxidant.

USED IN: *Vegetable oil, meat products, potato sticks, chicken soup base, chewing gum.*

Retards the spoilage of fats and oils. It is often used with **BHA** and **BHT** because of the synergistic effect these additives have in retarding rancidity. **Propyl gallate** has not been adequately tested, frequently is unnecessary, and should be avoided.

QUININE

FUNCTION: Flavoring

USED IN: *Tonic water, quinine water, bitter lemon.*

This drug can cure malaria and is used as a bitter flavoring in a few soft drinks. There is a slight chance that **quinine** may cause birth defects, so pregnant women should avoid quinine-containing beverages and drugs. Very poorly tested.

SACCHARIN

FUNCTION: Synthetic sweetener.

USED IN: *"Diet" products.*

Saccharin is 350 times sweeter than sugar and 10 times sweeter than cyclamate. Studies have not shown that saccharin helps people lose weight. Since 1951 tests have indicated that saccharin causes cancer. In 1977 the FDA proposed that saccharin be banned. Be wise—avoid **saccharin.**

SALT (SODIUM CHLORIDE)

FUNCTION: Flavoring.

USED IN: *Most processed foods; soup, potato chips, crackers.*

Salt is used liberally in many processed foods. Other additives contribute additional sodium. A diet high in sodium may cause high blood pressure, which increases the risk of heart attack and stroke. Everyone should eat less salt; avoid salty processed foods, use salt sparingly, enjoy other seasonings.

SODIUM NITRATE, SODIUM NITRITE

FUNCTION: Preservative, coloring, flavoring.

USED IN: *Bacon, ham, frankfurters, luncheon meats, smoked fish, corned beef.*

Nitrite can lead to the formation of small amounts of potent cancer-causing chemicals (nitrosamines), particularly in fried bacon. Nitrite is tolerated in foods because it can prevent the growth of bacteria that cause botulism poisoning. Nitrite also stabilizes the red color in cured meat and gives a characteristic flavor. Companies should find safer methods of preventing botulism. Meanwhile, *don't bring home the bacon.* **Sodium nitrate** is used in dry cured meat, because it slowly breaks down into nitrite.

SUCROSE (SUGAR)

FUNCTION: Sweetener.

USED IN: *Table sugar, sweetened foods.*

Sucrose, ordinary table sugar, occurs naturally in fruit, sugar cane, and sugar beets. Americans consume about 125 pounds of refined sugar per year. Sugar makes up about one-sixth of the average diet, but contains no vitamins, minerals, or protein. Sugar and sweetened foods may taste good and supply energy, but most people eat too much of them. Unless you enjoy large dentist bills and a large waistline, you should eat much less sugar.*

Hints for Good Health and Weight Loss

The Sensible Diet is based on *systematic undereating.* In other words, don't get up from the table hungry, but at the same time don't overstuff yourself. Most of us have been conditioned since childhood to eat everything on our plates. We were constantly reminded by our parents that people were starving throughout the world, and we were wasting food. Guilt (and in some cases obesity) was often the result of this early message to "clean our plates," compelling us to overeat into adulthood, even though we might not be hungry or feel hungry. Some simple solutions to the clean-your-plate syndrome are: first, serve smaller portions; second, if you're no longer hungry, put leftovers in the refrigerator and eat them the following day.

Eat a well-balanced breakfast, well-balanced lunch, and a *light* dinner. Recommended weight loss: *approximately one to two pounds per week, but not more.* (See the following suggestions for Controlling Eating Environments.)

Cook as little as possible. Cooking destroys many of the nutrients in food. Eat fruits and vegetables raw, or make your own raw vegetable and fruit juices. If you don't have a juicer, you can buy fresh juices at your local health food store. Another possibility is to steam your vegetables. Do not fry your food. Broil, bake or steam it instead.

Chew your food thoroughly. If you're pressed for time, you're better off skipping a meal than eating it in a hurry. If you're trying to lose weight, keep in mind that good chewing increases assimilation of nutrients in the intestinal tract and makes you feel satisfied with a smaller amount of food.

The following is a list of suggestions for controlling eating habits while on a weight-reduction protocol. It is from the book *Food Habit Management* by Julie Waltz,[32] with the addition of a few of my own suggestions in italics.

Controlling Eating Environments*

CONTROLLING YOUR HOME ENVIRONMENT
- Eat at the kitchen or dining room table.
- Eat sitting down.
- Eat without reading or watching TV.
- Keep tempting foods out of sight ("out of sight, out of mind").
- Make tempting foods hard to reach.
- Make tempting foods bothersome to prepare.
- Have low-calorie foods ready to eat, in sight, and easy to reach.
- Give other family members their own snack food cupboard.
- When possible, stay out of the kitchen.

CONTROLLING YOUR WORK ENVIRONMENT
- Do not eat at your desk.
- Do not keep tempting food in your desk drawers.
- Take pre-packaged meals, snacks and treats to work.
- Carry no change for vending machines.
- Eat a planned snack before leaving work.
- *Jump rope, or take a walk instead of having a high calorie snack during a work break.*
- Plan your cafeteria order in advance.
- Bring just enough money to pay for your planned order.

DAILY FOOD MANAGEMENT
SHOPPING
- Do not shop when hungry.
- Do not shop when tired.
- Shop from a specific list.
- Don't buy your favorite varieties of high-calorie foods.
- Buy small packages of hard-to-resist foods.
- *Carry your groceries to the car instead of using a cart.*

* Reprinted by permission of Northwest Learning Associates, Inc.

PREPARATION

- Prepare food when your control is highest.
- Prepare lunches and snacks when another meal is being cooked.
- Use a quarter teaspoon for tasting.
- If you prepare more than one meal at a time, cook each portion in a separate pot and freeze the extra portions immediately.
- When baking for others, don't bake your favorites.
- Use smaller containers for mixing, baking, and cooking.

CLEANUP AND LEFTOVERS

- Pour water, salt, sugar, or hot sauce over unwanted leftovers.
- Package and label usable leftovers for a specific meal or snack.
- Freeze containers of leftovers for soups or stews.
- If there is not good use for a leftover food, throw it out!

CONTROLLING YOUR MEALTIME ENVIRONMENT

- Don't keep serving bowls at the table.
- Use smaller plates, bowls, and glasses.
- Leave a little bit of food on your plate.
- Remove the plate as soon as you have finished eating.
- Politely refuse offers of extra food.
- *Don't feel that you have to eat everything on your plate.*

EATING SLOWLY: REDUCING EFFICIENCY

- Put the utensil or food down between bites.
- Cut food as it is needed.
- *Chew food slowly and thoroughly.*
- Swallow your food before preparing the next bite.
- Stop eating for a minute once or twice during the meal.
- Allow for second servings by making each serving one-half of the original amount.
- Serve yourself one food item at a time.

SNACK CONTROL: DELAYED EATING RESPONSE

- Wait 20 minutes before eating in response to an impulsive urge to eat.
- Replace eating with a different activity *such as jumping rope, jogging, tennis, or stretching.*
- Do something that can't or won't be combined with food, preferably something which involves using your mouth and hands at the same time such as playing an instrument or talking on the telephone.
- Do something you particularly like to do.
- Do a little task or a small part of a bigger job.
- Brush your teeth and use mouthwash.
- Move away from the sight, smell or sound of tempting food.

SNACK CONTROL: FOOD SUBSTITUTIONS

- Use an unrewarding snack food.
- Precede snacks with a large glass of water.
- For sweet cravings: eat a dill pickle first to reduce the desire for sweets. *If you still have a desire for sweets, eat a fresh apple or ¼ of a cantaloupe.*
- For cheese cravings: eat a little of a very rich, strongly flavored cheese.
- Keep enjoyable low-calorie snack foods available.
- Pre-package high-calorie foods in small amounts.
- Pre-package food "Emergency Kits" for times when you are upset, depressed, lonely, angry or likely to eat out of control.

SOCIAL EATING: RESTAURANTS, BUFFETS, CAFETERIAS, HOME ENTERTAINING BASICS

- Don't arrive hungry; eat something before you leave home.
- Plan a control strategy.
- Eat the best and skip the rest!
- Pour salt, pepper or sugar over foods you want to leave uneaten.
- Share orders of high-calorie items with someone.

- If you are still hungry after the meal, wait at least 20 minutes before asking for more.
- Use alcoholic beverages sparingly before the meal.
- Wear an outfit with a not-too-roomy waistband.

RESTAURANTS
- Order a la carte.
- Order according to the length of time you will spend in the restaurant and according to whether or not you will be eating again soon.
- Order some vegetables or a salad to be brought to the table right away.
- Ask to have the salad dressing brought in a separate dish.
- Ask for a "doggy bag" to take the extra food home.

BUFFETS AND CAFETERIAS
- Eat a plate of salad first.
- Use a serving spoon for servings; use a half-teaspoon for tastes.
- Use a salad plate instead of a dinner plate.
- Cover half of your dinner plate with green salad.
- Ask someone to get your food, and you get theirs.

ENTERTAINING AT HOME
- Use cookbooks with reduced calorie recipes.
- Use single-serving foods, like chicken breasts as opposed to casseroles, lasagna, etc. Leftovers may be a problem.
- Prepare a specific amount per person.
- Keep appetizers more than one arm's distance away.
- Take a serving of only one or two items at a time.
- Immediately place all mixing bowls and utensils in soapy water before licking them clean.
- Ask someone else to put the food items away while you clean up another room.[32] *

Menu for the Sensible Diet

The Sensible Diet Menu is based largely on my own personal eating habits, although, because of the amount of physical exercise I engage in each day, I tend to consume, as well as expend, far more calories than most people. Several choices are given for each meal to vary according to your own preferences. Feel free to experiment with the recommended foods discussed earlier in the chapter, creating or modifying your own recipes to fit the Sensible Diet approach. (Recipes for all items marked with an asterisk (*), plus a few more, will be found at the end of the chapter.)

BREAKFAST

CHOICE I
*Fresh fruit salad (bananas, grapes, apples, etc.) with yogurt or low-fat cottage cheese
    or
*Cantaloupe and cottage cheese delight
1 or 2 slices whole wheat toast
(Optional for those who need an extra boost in the morning: 2 oz. low-fat cheese melted on toast.)
To drink: Water with a squeeze of lemon juice, herb tea or fresh fruit juice.

CHOICE II
*Uncooked rolled oats and Post Grapenuts mixed together with fresh fruit.
    or
*Cooked natural grain cereal
To drink: Juice of 3 fresh oranges

CHOICE III
*Fool's Delight
1 slice whole wheat, rye or Pita bread
To drink: 8 oz. glass of any of the following juices: orange, tomato, grapefruit, pineapple or vegetable juice mixture
Remember to limit eggs to 3–5 per week.

CHOICE IV
*David Luna's Energy Drink

LUNCH

CHOICE I
Tuna sandwich on whole wheat or Pita bread with lettuce, tomato, alfalfa sprouts and sunflower seeds
or
*Luna's Tuna Salad
Dressing: Natural herb dressing or lemon juice
To drink: Fresh carrot juice, herb tea or Perrier water

CHOICE II
Baked potato topped with plain low-fat yogurt and Spike seasoning
Small mixed green salad with dressings as above
To drink: Herb tea

CHOICE III
*Pita sandwich
or
*Spinach and mushroom salad
1 slice whole wheat bread
To drink: 8 oz. skim milk or 6 oz. low-fat kefir (drink similar to liquid yogurt)

CHOICE IV
Bowl of any of the following soups:
*Mother's vegetable soup; lentil, or split pea soup (without meat)
Small bowl of steamed rice (if not included in soup)
4 unsalted whole wheat crackers
To drink: Spring water

DINNER

CHOICE I
*Steamed vegetables with melted cheese
One serving brown rice or 1 cob of corn

CHOICE II
*One fresh halibut steak or filet of sole (broiled or baked)
Small salad with recommended dressings

CHOICE III
*Eggplant parmesan
One serving brown rice

CHOICE IV
*Mother's vegetable soup mixed with brown rice

To drink with any of the above choices: Perrier or Poland water with a wedge of lime.
Lunch and dinner choices are interchangeable.

Recipes

All recipes serve 1, unless otherwise indicated.

BREAKFAST

FRESH FRUIT SALAD

2 or 3 fresh fruits in season, sliced
2 Tbsp. raisins or currants
2 Tbsp. sunflower seeds
1/2 cup plain low-fat yogurt or low-fat cottage cheese

Place fruit in small bowl. Toss with yogurt or add scoop of cottage cheese. Sprinkle with raisins and seeds. Enjoy!

CANTALOUPE AND COTTAGE CHEESE DELIGHT

1/2 cantaloupe, sliced lengthwise and seeded
1/2 cup low-fat cottage cheese
1 tsp. bran

Fill cantaloupe half with cottage cheese. Sprinkle with bran and dig in.

COOKED NATURAL GRAIN CEREAL

1 cup water
1/2 cup Quaker Whole Wheat Hot Natural Cereal
1/2 cup rolled oats
1/2 cup Post Grapenuts
2 Tbsp. raisins
1/4 cup unsweetened applesauce or strawberries

Bring water to boil in small saucepan. Add cereals. Cook for 5 minutes. Stir in raisins and cook 1-2 minutes longer. Serve topped with applesauce or strawberries.

ROLLED OATS AND GRAPENUTS

1 cup uncooked rolled oats
2-3 Tbsp. Post Grapenuts
1 tsp. Miller's Bran
1 Tbsp. unsalted sunflower seeds (optional)
1/2 cup low-fat or non-fat milk

Choice of 1 of the following fruits as sweetener:
1/2 banana
1-2 Tbsp. raisins
1 fresh peach, sliced
4-6 strawberries
2-3 dried figs
2-3 prunes

Place oats in small bowl. Top with remaining ingredients. Pour on the milk and start to munch.

FOOL'S DELIGHT

2 large eggs
1/2 tomato, coarsely chopped
1/4 large bell pepper, chopped
3 large mushrooms, sliced
1/8-1/4 onion, finely grated
2 oz. low-fat or skim cheese, sliced thin

Beat eggs. Pour into preheated teflon pan or other frying pan to which a small amount of vegetable oil has been added. Cook for about 1 minute, stirring constantly until eggs just begin to congeal. Stir in vegetables, cover and simmer for about 3 minutes. Place cheese on top, cover again and cook 1 or 2 minutes longer, until cheese is melted and eggs begin to puff. Do not overcook. Fold over and enjoy.

DAVID LUNA ENERGY DRINK

12 oz. orange juice
1 banana or 4–6 strawberries (fresh or frozen unsweetened)
1 tsp. fresh wheat germ
1 Tbsp. bran
1 tsp. brewer's yeast
6–10 almonds, or 2 Tbsp. unsalted sunflower seeds

If you don't want to take the time to sit down and eat breakfast, try this: Place juice in blender. Add remaining ingredients. If you would like to add a raw egg from time to time, do so, but remember the limit is 3–5 eggs per week. You might also try using a different base, such as apple or pineapple juice; low-fat, non-fat, or powdered milk. Experiment with different combinations until you find the energy drink you like best.

LUNCH

PITA SANDWICH

1 slice whole wheat pita bread
2–4 slices skim or low-fat cheese
2 slices tomato
1 leaf Romaine lettuce
1/4 cup alfalfa sprouts

Cut pita bread to create a pocket for sandwich. Add cheese. Place sandwich in 350° oven until cheese melts (about 5–10 minutes). Remove from oven and add tomato, lettuce, and sprouts.

LUNA'S TUNA SALAD

4 leaves Romaine lettuce
3–5 fresh mushrooms, sliced
1 tomato, quartered
1/2 small zucchini, sliced
1/4 cup garbanzo beans
1 scoop of tuna, packed in water
1/4 cup alfalfa sprouts
1 Tbsp. pine nuts
Optional: 2 slices low-fat or skim cheese
Gayelord Houser's "Spike" Seasoning
Herb dressing or lemon juice

Combine all vegetables except alfalfa sprouts in small salad bowl. Top with scoop of tuna and sprinkle with sprouts and pine nuts. Add Spike seasoning, herb dressing, or lemon juice.

SPINACH AND MUSHROOM SALAD

1/2 bunch fresh spinach leaves
1/2 cup fresh mushrooms, sliced
1 tomato, quartered
1 hard boiled egg, sliced thin
2 Tbsp. unsalted sunflower seeds
Apple cider vinegar or herb dressing

Wash spinach leaves thoroughly. Add mushrooms, tomato, hard boiled egg, and sunflower seeds. Toss together with dressing and serve at once.

DINNER

STEAMED VEGETABLES WITH MELTED CHEESE

3 or more fresh vegetables, cut in large pieces (choose from list at beginning of this chapter)
2 oz. skim cheese, sliced thin or grated
1 cup cooked brown rice

Steam vegetables until just cooked, but not too soft. Transfer to a bake-and-serve dish. Top with cheese. Bake at 375° for 10 minutes, or until cheese melts. Serve with brown rice. Easy, beautiful and delicious!

EGGPLANT PARMESAN

1 large can whole tomatoes
1 can (29 oz.) tomato sauce
1 can (6 oz.) tomato paste
3–4 bay leaves
1 medium eggplant
1 medium bell pepper
1 medium onion
2 celery stalks
1/2 lb. fresh mushrooms
8 oz. low-fat or skim cheese

Chop pepper, onion, celery, and mushrooms and mix with tomato sauce, tomato paste, bay leaves and whole tomatoes. Simmer sauce about 3 hours. Meanwhile, grate the cheese and boil eggplant for about 20–25 minutes. When soft, cool and cut into slices. Place in baking dish, add half of the sauce and half of the grated cheese. Repeat with remaining eggplant, sauce, and top with cheese. Bake 1 hour at 350°. Variations: Substitute zucchini or other squash for eggplant. Serves 4.

FRESH BAKED HALIBUT

1 fresh halibut steak
1 tsp. herb seasoning
Juice of 1/2 lemon (or 3 Tbsp. dry white wine)

Place halibut steak in large baking dish. Season with herb seasoning. Add lemon juice or wine. Bake at 350° for 20 minutes. (Fish may also be broiled with the same seasonings.) Serve with a small salad.

MOTHER'S VEGETABLE SOUP

10 cups water
3 tomatoes, sliced
1 zucchini, sliced
1 onion, sliced
2 potatoes, sliced unpeeled
corn from 2 cobs
1/2 small cabbage, sliced
3 carrots, sliced unpeeled
3 celery stalks, coarsely chopped
2 tsp. sea salt or herb seasoning
2 cups cooked brown rice (optional)

Bring water to boil in large pot. Add vegetables and seasoning. Cook over low flame for 1 hour. Add cooked rice, if desired, and serve. Fantastic!! Serves 4.

SNACKS

FRESH APPLE AND YOGURT

1 apple, unpeeled, sliced in quarters
1/2 cup plain low-fat yogurt

Dip apple slices into yogurt and munch away.

PITA BREAD AND APPLE SAUCE

1/2 slice Pita bread
3 Tbsp. unsweetened applesauce
1 Tbsp. unsalted sunflower seeds

Spread applesauce over bread. Sprinkle with sunflower seeds for a yummy treat anytime.

TRAIL MIX

Raw, unsalted almonds
Pumpkin seeds
Sunflower seeds
Unsulfured raisins

Mix all ingredients in equal amounts. Trail mix is not only delicious, but also high in calories, so eat sparingly.

RAW VEGETABLE JUICE

Recommended combinations:
Carrot, celery and beet
Carrot, celery and cucumber
Tomato, celery and parsley

Raw vegetable juice can also be purchased at most health food stores in pint or quart containers. Do not buy it if it is more than one day old, as raw vegetable juices tend to oxidize very rapidly. If possible, buy a juicer to insure freshness.

UNSALTED CRACKERS WITH SKIM OR LOW-FAT CHEESE

FRESH FRUIT

5. Vitamins

What About Vitamins?

At the moment, vitamin supplementation is a very controversial subject. On the one hand, orthodox medicine contends that all the necessary nutrients can be derived from a "well-balanced diet." On the other hand, there is a growing opinion among those who practice preventive medicine that food supplements are not only vital, but imperative. Who's right?

Let's examine the issue. Fifty percent of the American population is malnourished. Senator George McGovern stated recently that malnutrition should refer not only to underconsumption and poverty, but to overconsumption and faulty diet at all economic levels.

The argument given by most doctors and dieticians is that all nutrients can be obtained from a "well-balanced diet." That may be true, but how many people eat a well-balanced diet? Most don't even know what it is, and many of those who do, don't adhere to it.

Another argument is that a hundred years ago, our ancestors didn't require any vitamin supplementation, so why should we? A hundred years ago most people in this country ate wholesome foods which were naturally grown on their own farms without the aid of chemical fertilizers. A hundred years ago, they ate fresh fruits and vegetables from their own gardens without toxic sprays. A hundred years ago, they ate no processed or refined foods. A hundred years ago, they ate no processed or depleted foods. A hundred years ago, foods were not grown on depleted soils and were not denatured and devitalized by processing and refining. A hundred years ago, foods were free from DDT, synthetic estrogenic hormones, preservatives, insecticides, tetracycline, testosterone and other chemicals and drugs.

Many fruits and vegetables are picked in an unripened state so they won't spoil while being transported, thereby decreasing nutritional value. During transportation many of our foods are exposed to freezing and oxidation, resulting in nutrient loss. Wheat germ, for example, stays fresh for about seven to ten days after it's processed. Shortly thereafter, it begins to oxidize and become rancid. Even storing wheat germ in cold temperatures doesn't prevent it from oxidizing or becoming rancid, but only slows down the process. Most Americans who eat wheat germ regularly are unaware that it's rancid. Fresh wheat germ has a sweet, delicious taste. Rancid wheat germ tastes bitter and acrid. After a while, most people assume that the bitter aftertaste of wheat germ is an inherent characteristic. Freshly milled wheat germ is very difficult to buy unless you're fortunate enough to live near a mill where it's processed or a good health store that sells packages dated for freshness. If you purchase wheat germ and find that it is rancid, return it.

At the present time, about 45% of the calories in the American diet comes from fats. This includes 17% in the form of fats that are added back to foods during the cooking process, such as the deep frying of donuts. Sugar is responsible for another 17% of our calories. This means that more than a third of our caloric intake comes from foods that contain virtually no vitamins or minerals. Refined white flour is another culprit, constituting 11% of our caloric intake while at the same time denying us the valuable nutrients that are substantially removed during the heavy milling process. We need to ask ourselves how we can get all the vitamins and minerals we need when 45% of the calories we consume are derived from fat, sugar and foods stripped of much of their nutritional value through processing.

Cooked foods also lose much of their nutritional value by the time they reach the table. Dr. Paavo Airola has gone so far as to say that cooked food is dead food.[1] I'm not against cooking food; however, I am aware that most of us have a tendency to overcook. Therefore, we should undercook as much as possible, and eat most fruits and vegetables raw whenever possible.

These are just a few of the reasons why eating a "well-balanced diet" in this day and age may not be sufficient. The Food and Nutrition Board, National Academy of Sciences, National Research Council, provides Recommended Daily Dietary Allowances designed for the maintenance of good nutrition of practically all healthy people in the U.S.A. Refer to their recommendations (Figs. 5–1 and 5–2) to determine your own requirements.

If you should decide to take vitamins to supplement your diet, keep in mind that they should be taken *with a meal* for better absorption and assimilation. Also, there are two different types of vitamins: fat-soluble and water-soluble.

The fat-soluble vitamins consist of vitamins A, D, E and K. These vitamins are generally retained in the body and therefore should not be taken in large doses. The water-soluble vitamins consist of the B-complex vitamins and vitamin C. These are retained for short periods, if at all, and are water-dispersable. In other words, they're dissolved in water, whereas fat-soluble vitamins are dissolved in fat. Since there is no universal agreement on recommended doses, my advice is to take moderate amounts of both the fat-soluble and the water-soluble vitamins, should you decide to supplement. Also keep in mind that no two people have identical requirements, so that what seems appropriate for one person may not be right for another.

All vitamins and minerals work synergistically—in other words, they work together. Unless you know for certain that you have a specific vitamin deficiency, do *not*, for example, start taking an inordinant amount of the B-complex vitamins on an independent basis. To do so may create an imbalance. Also, many people have a tendency to self prescribe as soon as they read an article or report about a condition or disease which they feel is pertinent to them. This may not be in your best interests, so don't be gullible and influenced by everything that you read or hear, particularly if it is from an unreliable source.

FIG. 5–1

RECOMMENDED DIETARY ALLOWANCES (RDA), Revised 1980

Age (years)	Weight (kg)	Weight (lbs)	Height (cm)	Height (in)	Protein (g)	Vitamin A (RE)[a]	Vitamin B (µg)[b]	Vitamin E (mg α TE)[c]	Vitamin C (mg)	Thiamin (mg)	Riboflavin (mg)	Niacin (mg NE)[d]	Vitamin B_6 (mg)	Folacin (µg)	Vitamin B_{12} (µg)	Calcium (mg)	Phosphorus (mg)	Magnesium (mg)	Iron (mg)	Zinc (mg)	Iodine (µg)
Infants																					
0.0–0.5	6	13	60	24	kg x 2.2	420	10	3	35	0.3	0.4	6	0.3	30	0.5[e]	360	240	50	10	3	40
0.5–1.0	9	20	71	28	kg x 2.0	400	10	4	35	0.5	0.6	8	0.6	45	1.5	540	360	70	15	5	50
Children																					
1–3	13	29	90	35	23	400	10	5	45	0.7	0.8	9	0.9	100	2.0	800	800	150	15	10	70
4–6	20	44	112	44	30	500	10	6	45	0.9	1.0	11	1.3	200	2.5	800	800	200	10	10	90
7–10	28	62	132	52	34	700	10	7	45	1.2	1.4	16	1.6	300	3.0	800	800	250	10	10	120
Males																					
11–14	45	99	157	62	45	1000	10	8	50	1.4	1.6	18	1.8	400	3.0	1200	1200	350	18	15	150
15–18	66	145	176	69	56	1000	10	10	60	1.4	1.7	18	2.0	400	3.0	1200	1200	400	18	15	150
19–22	70	154	177	70	56	1000	7.5	10	60	1.5	1.7	19	2.2	400	3.0	800	800	350	10	15	150
23–50	70	154	178	70	56	1000	5	10	60	1.4	1.6	18	2.2	400	3.0	800	800	350	10	15	150
51 +	70	154	178	70	56	1000	5	10	60	1.2	1.4	16	2.2	400	3.0	800	800	350	10	15	150
Females																					
11–14	46	101	157	62	46	800	10	8	50	1.1	1.3	15	1.8	400	3.0	1200	1200	300	18	15	150
15–18	55	120	163	64	46	800	10	8	60	1.1	1.3	14	2.0	400	3.0	1200	1200	300	18	15	150
19–22	55	120	163	64	44	800	7.5	8	60	1.1	1.3	14	2.0	400	3.0	800	800	300	18	15	150
23–50	55	120	163	64	44	800	5	8	60	1.0	1.2	13	2.0	400	3.0	800	800	300	18	15	150
51 +	55	120	163	64	44	800	5	8	60	1.0	1.2	13	2.0	400	3.0	800	800	300	10	15	150
Pregnant					+ 30	+ 200	+ 5	+ 2	+ 20	+ 0.4	+ 0.3	+ 2	0.6	+ 400	+ 1.0	+ 400	+ 400	+ 150	f	+ 5	+ 25
Lactating					+ 20	+ 400	+ 5	+ 3	40	+ 0.5	+ 0.5	+ 5	+ 0.5	+ 100	+ 1.0	+ 400	+ 400	+ 150	f	+ 10	+ 50

The allowances are intended to provide for individual variations among most normal, healthy people in the United States under usual environmental stresses. They were designed for the maintenance of good nutrition. Diets should be based on a variety of common foods in order to provide other nutrients for which human requirements have been less well defined.

[a] Retinol equivalents. 1 Retinol equivalent = 1 µg retinol or 6 µg carotene.

[b] As cholecalciferol. 10 µg cholecalciferol + 400 IU vitamin D

[c] Tocopherol equivalents. 1 mg d-α-tocopherol = 1 α TE

[d] 1 NE (niacin equivalent) is equal to 1 mg of niacin or 60 mg of dietary tryptophan.

[e] The RDA for vitamin B_{12} in infants is based on average concentration of the vitamin in human milk. The allowances after weaning are based on energy intake (as recommended by the American Academy of Pediatrics) and consideration of other factors such as intestinal absorption.

[f] The increased requirement during pregnancy cannot be met by the iron content of habitual American diets nor by the existing iron stores of many women; therefore the use of 30–60 mg of supplemental iron is recommended. Iron needs during lactation are not substantially different from those of nonpregnant women, but continued supplementation of the mother for 2–3 months after parturition is advisable in order to replenish stores depleted by pregnancy.

RDA revised and published in 1980 by the Food and Nutrition Board. National Academy of Sciences/ National Research Council. Washington. D.C.

FIG. 5–2

ESTIMATED SAFE AND ADEQUATE DAILY DIETARY INTAKES OF ADDITIONAL SELECTED VITAMINS AND MINERALS

Because there is less information on which to base allowances, these figures are not given in the main table of the RDA and are provided here in the form of ranges of recommended intakes.

	Vitamins			Trace Elements[a]						Electrolytes		
Age (years)	Vitamin K (µg)	Biotin (µg)	Pantothenic Acid (mg)	Copper (mg)	Manganese (mg)	Fluoride (mg)	Chromium (mg)	Selenium (mg)	Molybdenum (mg)	Sodium (mg)	Potassium (mg)	Chloride (mg)
Infants												
0–0.5	12	35	2	0.5–0.7	0.5–0.7	0.1–0.5	0.01–0.04	0.01–0.04	0.03–0.06	115–350	350–925	275–700
0.5–1	10–20	50	3	0.7–1.0	0.7–1.0	0.2–1.0	0.02–0.06	0.02–0.06	0.04–0.08	250–750	425–1275	400–1200
Children and adolescents												
1–3	15–30	65	3	1.0–1.5	1.0–1.5	0.5–1.5	0.02–0.08	0.02–0.08	0.05–0.1	325–975	550–1650	500–1500
4–6	20–40	85	3–4	1.5–2.0	1.5–2.0	1.0–2.5	0.03–0.12	0.03–0.12	0.06–0.15	450–1350	775–2325	700–2100
7–10	30–60	120	4–5	2.0–2.5	2.0–3.0	1.5–2.5	0.05–0.2	0.05–0.2	0.1 –0.3	600–1800	1000–3000	925–2775
11 +	50–100	100–200	4–7	2.0–3.0	2.5–5.0	1.5–2.5	0.05–0.2	0.05–0.2	0.15–0.5	900–2700	1525–4575	1400–4200
Adults	70–140	100–200	4–7	2.0–3.0	2.5–5.0	1.5–4.0	0.05–0.2	0.05–0.2	0.15–0.5	1100–3300	1875–5625	1700–5100

[a] Since the toxic levels for many trace elements may be only several times usual intakes, the upper levels for the trace elements given in this table should not be habitually exceeded.

From Recommended Dietary Allowances, revised 1980. Food and Nutrition Board, National Academy of Sciences/National Research Council, Washington, D.C.

Are Iron Supplements Necessary?

The answer to this question depends on one's particular needs and whether or not the diet is meeting those needs. There are instances where increased iron requirements simply cannot be met by ordinary diets. It has been well established that during periods of growth such as infancy, childhood, adolescence, and pregnancy, there is an increased absorption of iron, which may lead to iron-deficiency anemia. Also, most women, from the onset of menstruation through menopause, tend to be iron deficient.

Iron-deficiency anemia is a condition in which the red blood cells contain less hemoglobin (an oxygen carrier in the blood) and lose their ability to hold oxygen. This condition can be detected by a simple blood test. If in doubt, check with your physician, particularly if fatigue is a constant symptom.

The American diet provides only about 5–6 mg. of iron per 1000 k calories. This is fine as long as one is an adult male. An adult male, whose RDA is 10 mg. and who eats about 2,400–2,500 k calories, has no trouble meeting his RDA. However, a woman, whose RDA is 18 mg., and who may eat less than 2,000 k calories per day, will undoubtedly have more difficulty meeting these requirements.

Following is a list of foods that are rich sources of iron:

FIG. 5–3

SOURCES OF IRON

Food	Approximate Amount	Iron (mg)
Oysters (raw)	1 cup	13.2
Bran flakes (40% bran) (added thiamin and iron)	1 cup	12.3
Prune juice (canned or bottled)	1 cup	10.5
Dried apricots	1 cup	8.2
Black walnuts	1 cup	7.6
Almonds	1 cup	6.7
Raisins (seedless)	1 cup	5.8
Dates (pitted)	1 cup	5.3
Clams (raw)	3 ounces	5.2
Navy beans	1 cup	4.9
Red kidney beans	1 cup	4.6
Lettuce	1 head	4.4
Lima beans	1 cup	4.3
Split peas (dry)	1 cup	4.2
Spinach (cooked)	1 cup	4.0
Barley (uncooked)	1 cup	4.0
Cowpeas or blackeye peas	1 cup	3.4
Dandelion greens (cooked)	1 cup	3.2
Green peas (cooked)	1 cup	2.9
Spaghetti in tomato sauce with cheese (canned)	1 cup	2.8
Beet greens (leaves and stems)	1 cup	2.8

Food	Approximate Amount	Iron (mg)
Pecans (halves)	1 cup	2.6
Shrimp	3 ounces	2.6
Sardines	3 ounces	2.5
White rice (enriched)	1 cup	1.8
Avocados	1 avocado	1.8
Brussels sprouts	1 cup	1.7
Tuna	3 ounces	1.6
Whole wheat bread	2 slices	1.6
Apple juice (bottled or canned)	1 cup	1.5
Rolled oats or oatmeal	1 cup	1.4
Broccoli (cooked)	1 stalk	1.4
½ Chicken breast	3.3 ounces	1.3
Macaroni (enriched)	1 cup	1.3
Mushrooms (canned)	1 cup	1.2
Eggs	1 egg	1.1
Ocean perch	3 ounces	1.1
Swordfish	3 ounces	1.1
Tomatoes	1 tomato	0.9

Effect of Cooking

Cooking methods have an important effect on the amount of iron in the diet. Simmering or sautéing in an unenameled iron skillet, for example, can triple the iron content of foods, even in the short time it takes to scramble an egg. The iron content of 100 gm. of spaghetti sauce simmered in a glass pot is only 3 mg. compared to 87 mg. when it is cooked in an iron utensil.

Conversely, iron already concentrated in the skins of foods such as potatoes and carrots is often lost into cooking water which is then discarded. Don't peel your vegetables, since that's where most of the nutritional value lies. Steam rather than boil, and cook vegetables for shorter periods of time and in less water.

Natural Versus Synthetic Vitamins

This is still yet another controversial issue. Most doctors address this issue by saying, "A vitamin is a vitamin." Others tend to disagree.

A natural vitamin is one which derives its ingredients from a natural source. A synthetic vitamin, manufactured in a laboratory, is identical to a natural vitamin found in foods. The body cannot tell the difference and gets the same benefits from either source. Statements to the effect that "Nature cannot be imitated" and "Natural vitamins have the essence of life" are without meaning.[2]

For those of you who are interested in being able to differentiate between a natural and a synthetic vitamin, I've included a chart to show you the difference (Fig. 5–4). Compare this information with the sources listed on the vitamin bottle.

Remember, all synthetic vitamins are "organic" when the most liberal interpretation of that word is applied: namely, the substance has present in its molecular structure the element carbon. Scientifically speaking, that is all that is needed to qualify a substance as organic.

FIG. 5-4

SOURCES OF NATURAL AND SYNTHETIC VITAMINS

Item:	If source given is:	It is:
Vitamin A	Fish oils	Natural
	Acetate	Synthetic
	Palmitate-lemon grass	Synthetic
	Water dispersible	Synthetic
Vitamin B$_1$	Yeast	Natural
	Thiamine mononitrate	Synthetic
	Thiamine hydrochloride	Synthetic
Vitamin B$_2$	Yeast	Natural
	Riboflavin	Synthetic
Vitamin B$_6$	Yeast	Natural
	Pyridoxine hydrochloride	Synthetic
Vitamin B$_{12}$	Yeast	Natural
	Streptomycin fermentation	Crystalline
	Cobalamin concentrate	Crystalline
Folic Acid	Yeast	Natural
	Peroyglutamic acid	Synthetic
Pantothenic Acid	Yeast	Natural
	Calcium pantothenate	Synthetic
Choline	Soy beans	Natural
	Choline bitartrate	Synthetic
Biotin	Liver	Natural
	d-biotin	Synthetic
Nicotinic Acid	Yeast	Natural
	Niacin	Synthetic

Item:	If source given is:	It is:
Niacin	Yeast	Natural
	Niacinamide	Synthetic
Vitamin C	Citrus, rose hips, acerola berries	Natural (but fortified)
	Ascorbic acid	Synthetic
Vitamin D	Fish oil	Natural
	Irradiated ergosterol	Synthetic
	Calciferol	Synthetic
	Activated yeast	Synthetic
Vitamin E	Mixed tocopherols	Natural
	Wheat germ oil	Natural
	d'Alpha tocopherol	Crystalline
	d'l Alpha tocopherol	Synthetic
	Water dispersible	Crystalline
Vitamin K	Alfalfa	Natural
	Menadione	Synthetic

NATURAL: When the word natural is applied to a food supplement it should mean that the ingredients in that supplement are derived from food concentration such as fish liver oil, yeast, etc.

CRYSTALLINE: A crystalline vitamin has its source in a natural food by means of distillation, heat, or solvents that have been isolated into a specific vitamin or amino acid.

SYNTHETIC: When a vitamin is put together in the laboratory by duplicating the exact molecular structure of a crystalline vitamin, the resulting product is a synthetic form of the vitamin.

The Vitamins: Sources and Functions

VITAMIN A

Also known as the anti-infective or anti-ophthalmic vitamin. Usually measured in U.S.P. units.

NATURAL SOURCES: Fresh fruits; carrots; squash; yams; tomatoes; broccoli; leafy green vegetables such as spinach, kale, collard greens, and turnip greens; milk; cheese; and fish-liver oils.

FUNCTIONS: Builds resistance to infections, especially of the respiratory tract. Helps maintain a healthy condition of the outer layers of many tissues and organs. Promotes new cell growth and healthy tissues. Permits formation of visual purple in the eye, counteracting night-blindness and weak eyesight. Promotes healthy skin. Essential for pregnancy and lactation.

VITAMIN B_1

Thiamine, Thiamine Chloride. Also known as the anti-neuritic or anti-beriberi vitamin. Generally expressed in milligrams (mg), occasionally in units. 333 units of B_1 equal only 1.0 mg.

NATURAL SOURCES: Brewer's yeast; wheat germ (only if fresh); wheat bran; whole grain cereals such as wheat, oats, and rice; seeds and nuts; beans; milk and milk products; and vegetables such as beets, potatoes, and leafy green vegetables; poultry and fish.

FUNCTIONS: Prevents beriberi (a dysfunction of the nervous system). Promotes growth. Essential for proper metabolism of carbohydrates and fats. Helps to maintain normal red blood count, improves circulation, and helps prevent fatigue.

VITAMIN B_2

Riboflavin. Measured in milligrams (mg).

NATURAL SOURCES: Milk; eggs; cheese; whole grains; brewer's yeast; fresh wheat germ; almonds; sunflower seeds; and leafy green vegetables.

FUNCTIONS: Helps the body obtain energy from carbohydrates and protein substances. Improves growth; essential for healthy eyes, skin and mouth.

VITAMIN B_3

Nicotinic Acid (Niacin). Niacinamide (Nicotinamide). The functions and deficiency symptoms of these members of the B-complex are similar. Niacinamide is more generally used since it minimizes the burning, flushing and itching of the skin that frequently occurs with nicotinic acid.

NATURAL SOURCES: Brewer's yeast; sunflower seeds; peanuts; brown rice; green vegetables; whole wheat products; and fish.

FUNCTIONS: Prevents pellagra (a condition characterized by an inflammation of the skin, mouth sores, diarrhea, and mental disorders.) Important for the proper functioning of nervous system. Promotes growth. Maintains normal function of the gastro-intestinal tract. Necessary for metabolism of sugar.

PANTOTHENIC ACID

A member of the B-complex family.

NATURAL SOURCES: Brewer's yeast; potatoes; peas; rice; bran; sunflower seeds; whole wheat products; poultry; and fish.

FUNCTIONS: Not clearly defined as yet. Helps in the building of body cells and maintaining normal skin, growth, and development of central nervous system. Required for synthesis of antibodies. Necessary for normal digestive processes.

VITAMIN B$_6$

Pyridoxine. Measured in milligrams (mg). If it is designated micrograms (mcg), remember that it requires 1000 micrograms to equal 1.0 milligram (mg).

NATURAL SOURCES: Brewer's yeast; bananas; avocados; whole grain cereals; soybeans; walnuts; milk; potatoes and sweet potatoes; cabbage; corn; cantaloupe; egg yolks; leafy green vegetables; green peppers; carrots; and peanuts. Pecans are an especially rich source. Raw foods contain more B$_6$ than cooked foods.

FUNCTIONS: Primarily concerned with protein and fat metabolism; prevents various nervous and skin disorders, such as acne. Involved in the production of antibodies which protect against bacterial invasions. Essential for the synthesis and proper action of DNA and RNA.

FOLIC ACID (Folacin)

A member of the B-complex family.

NATURAL SOURCES: Dark green leafy vegetables, asparagus; broccoli; navy beans; Irish potatoes; spinach; lettuce; brewer's yeast; mushrooms; nuts; and whole wheat products.

FUNCTIONS: Essential to the formation of red blood cells by its action on the bone marrow. Aids in protein metabolism and contributes to normal growth. Essential for healing processes. Helps to build antibodies to prevent and heal infections. Essential for the health of skin and hair.

CHOLINE

Measured in milligrams (mg).

NATURAL SOURCES: Egg yolks; green leafy vegetables; legumes; brewer's yeast; fresh wheat germ; milk; poultry; and fish; whole grain cereals.

FUNCTIONS: Regulates function of liver; necessary for normal fat metabolism. Minimizes excessive deposits of fat in liver.

INOSITOL

Measured in milligrams (mg).

NATURAL SOURCES: Citrus fruits; brewer's yeast; whole grains; and milk.

FUNCTIONS: Similar to that of choline.

BIOTIN

Member of the B-complex family.

NATURAL SOURCES: Best and richest natural source is brewer's yeast; also found in soybeans, nuts, and egg yolks. *Raw* egg white contains a factor that destroys biotin. Normally produced in the intestines if there is a sufficient amount of healthy intestinal flora (friendly bacteria).

FUNCTIONS: Growth-promoting factor. Possibly related to metabolism of fats and in the conversion of certain amino acids.

PABA

Para Amino Benzoic Acid.

NATURAL SOURCES: Brewer's yeast; whole grain products; milk;

eggs; yogurt; and fresh wheat germ. PABA is also synthesized by friendly bacteria in healthy intestines.

FUNCTIONS: A growth-promoting factor, possibly in conjunction with folic acid.

VITAMIN B₁₂

Commonly known as the "red vitamin." Cobalamin. Since it is so effective in small dosages, it is the only common vitamin generally expressed in micrograms (mg).

NATURAL SOURCES: Eggs; milk; cheese; fish; and poultry. B_{12} is not present to any measurable degree in plants, which means that strict vegetarians should supplement their diets with this vitamin.

FUNCTIONS: Helps in the formation and regeneration of red blood cells, thus helping to prevent anemia; promotes growth and increased appetite in children; a general tonic for adults; synthesis of DNA and RNA.

VITAMIN C

Ascorbic Acid, Cevitamic Acid. Usually expressed in milligrams (mg).

NATURAL SOURCES: All fresh fruits and vegetables. Particularly rich sources are citrus fruits; rose hips; berries; black currants; strawberries; cauliflower; cabbage; tomatoes; brussels sprouts; turnip greens; broccoli; collard greens; green bell peppers; melons; persimmons; guavas; and cherries.

FUNCTIONS: Prevents scurvy; necessary for healthy teeth, gums and bones; strengthens all connective tissue; promotes wound healing; helps promote capillary integrity and prevention of permeability, a very important factor in maintaining sound health and vigor; involved in the absorption and use of iron. Whether or not it helps to prevent and cure the common cold is still a controversial issue.

VITAMIN D

This vitamin exists in several forms. The most common (and equally effective) are ergocalciferol—vitamin D_2, and cholicalciferol—vitamin D_3. The D_2 is from a plant source; the D_3 comes from animal sources. Known as the "sunshine vitamin." Measured in U.S.P. units.

NATURAL SOURCES: Fish-liver oils; eggs; milk; sprouted seeds; mushrooms; sunflower seeds; and sunshine.

FUNCTIONS: Prevents rickets by regulating the use of calcium and phospherous in the body, making vitamin D necessary for the proper formation of bones and teeth. Very important in infancy and childhood. Synthesized in skin by activity of ultraviolet light.

VITAMIN E

Consists of Alpha, Beta, Delta and Gamma Tocopherols. Available in several different forms. Formerly measured by weight (mg)—now generally designated according to its biological activity in international units (IU).

NATURAL SOURCES: Vegetable oils such as wheat germ oil and soybean oil; whole wheat; leafy green vegetables; eggs; whole grain cereals; nuts; beans; and peas.

FUNCTIONS: One of its most important functions is that of an antioxidant, i.e., a compound that protects others from oxidation by being oxidized itself. Reduces the oxidation of vitamin A and polyunsaturated fatty acids. Evidence from animal studies shows that vitamin E provides some protection against lung damage from air pollutants such as nitrogen dioxide and ozone.[3] There is no evidence, however, that it improves athletic ability or is effective in the treatment of heart problems or muscular dystrophy.[4] Probably the most proliferated myth about vitamin E is that it improves sexual performance. Unfortunately, there is no evidence to support this.[5]

VITAMIN K

Menaquinone, Phyloquinone.

NATURAL SOURCES: Alfalfa; spinach; lettuce; kale; cabbage; cauliflower; egg yolks; and milk. Also synthesized in the intestinal tract with microorganisms.

FUNCTIONS: Essential for the production of prothrombin (a substance which aids the blood in clotting); important to liver function.

The Important Minerals

CALCIUM (Ca)

NATURAL SOURCES: Milk and dairy products; broccoli and leafy green vegetables, such as turnip and collard greens, kale, endive, lettuce, brussels sprouts, and dandelion greens; soybeans; sesame seeds; almonds; sunflower seeds; tortillas; and salmon.

FUNCTIONS: Builds and maintains bones and teeth; aids in the blood-clotting process (thrombin formation); muscle contraction; regulates heart rhythm; transmission of nerve impulses.

COBALT (Co)

NATURAL SOURCES: Milk; saltwater fish; leafy green vegetables; and poultry.

FUNCTIONS: Stimulant to production of red blood cells; component of vitamin B_{12}; necessary for normal growth and appetite.

COPPER (Cu)

NATURAL SOURCES: Whole grain cereals; almonds; mushrooms; cherries; beans; peas; saltwater fish; prunes; and raisins.

FUNCTIONS: Necessary for absorption and utilization of iron in the synthesis of hemoglobin; purine metabolism; metabolism of ascorbic acid.

FLUORINE (F)

NATURAL SOURCES: Fluoridated water: 1 ppm (parts per million).

FUNCTIONS: Essential for bone and tooth building. Increases resistance to osteoporosis.

IODINE (I)

NATURAL SOURCES: Iodized salt; seaweed and kelp (available in tablet form); fish; spinach; Swiss chard; artichokes; and collard greens.

FUNCTIONS: Necessary for proper function of thyroid gland; essential for proper growth; regulates the rate of energy metabolism.

IRON (Fe)

NATURAL SOURCES: Peas; beans; potatoes; poultry; prunes; raisins; brewer's yeast; spinach; lentils; peaches; apricots; bananas; whole grain cereals; and egg yolks (however only about 4% of the iron is absorbed in egg yolks).

FUNCTIONS: Required in the manufacture of hemoglobin; helps carry oxygen in the blood.

MAGNESIUM (Mg)

NATURAL SOURCES: Nuts; soybeans; whole grains; rice; peas; fish; and leafy green vegetables, such as spinach.

FUNCTIONS: Necessary for calcium and vitamin C metabolism; essential for normal functioning of nervous and muscular system; activates enzymes in carbohydrate metabolism.

MANGANESE (Mn)

NATURAL SOURCES: Whole grain cereals; nuts; brussels sprouts; spinach; apricots; oranges; grapefruit; peas; and fresh wheat germ.

FUNCTIONS: Activates various enzymes and other minerals; related to proper utilization of vitamines B_1 and E.

MOLYBDENUM (Mo)

NATURAL SOURCES: Peas; beans; whole grain cereals such as rice, millet, and buckwheat.

FUNCTIONS: Associated with carbohydrate metabolism.

PHOSPHOROUS (P)

NATURAL SOURCES: Cheese; peanuts; cod; halibut; whole grain cereals; seeds; nuts; eggs; and milk.

FUNCTIONS: Regulates the release of energy from the combustion or oxidation of carbohydrates, fats, and protein. Needed for normal bone and tooth structure. Interrelated with action of calcium and vitamin D. Calcium and phosphorous work together, so they must be present in proper balance to be effective.

POTASSIUM (K)

NATURAL SOURCES: Oranges; apricots; bananas; figs; potatoes (peel included); lima beans; fish and poultry.

FUNCTIONS: Involved in the release of energy, and in glycogen and protein synthesis; water balance; regular heart rhythm; muscle contraction and nerve irritability; acid-base balance; and involved with enzyme functions within the cells.

SODIUM (Na)

NATURAL SOURCES: See chart on Foods High in Salt (Fig. 4–6).

FUNCTIONS: Maintains the fluid and acid-base balance of the body; regulates nerve irritability and muscle contraction.

SULPHUR (S)

NATURAL SOURCES: Eggs; milk; cheese; celery; onions; string beans; radishes; and turnips.

FUNCTIONS: Vital to good skin, hair and nails.

ZINC (Zn)

NATURAL SOURCES: Peas; whole wheat cereals; oatmeal; fresh wheat germ; onions; eggs; milk; and fish.

FUNCTIONS: Helps normal tissue function; protein and carbohydrate metabolism. In addition to being an integral part of enzymes, zinc is required for the action of insulin.

6. Heart Disease and its Prevention

Heart disease is a killer—the number one killer in this country. Last year, according to the American Heart Association, there were almost 100,000 cardiovascular disease-related deaths in the United States. Of the 646,000 people who die of heart attacks each year, the first clinical indications of heart disease in over 60% of the males is sudden death.

You may be a prime candidate. If you're not sure what a prime candidate is, you can get some good clues from Dr. Richard T. Walden, a former professor at California Loma Linda University Medical Center.[1] Dr. Walden clearly spells out "How to Die Younger," with an all-too familiar regimen that thousands of Americans follow daily.

How to Die Younger*

1. OVEREAT

- Eat lots of fats, and be sure that most of these fats come animal sources or are hydrogenated.
- Get prosperous-looking and plump (for even being 10 percent overweight after age 35 may reduce your life expectancy by five years).
- Drink lots of whole milk, eat lots of cheese, whipped cream or whipped-cream substitutes, butter, ice cream (the latter goes well on frosted cakes or pies).
- Be sure to eat more than 4 eggs a week—it's the yolks that count.

*Reproduced by permission of Richard T. Walden, M.D., F.A.C.P., and Health Media Services, Loma Linda, California.

2. NEVER EXERCISE

- Use your car to go any distance more than a half block.

- Sit comfortably in front of the TV in the evenings—especially after a heavy meal.

- Get up only to walk to the refrigerator for more snacks during commercials. (With planning, even this exercise can be reduced if you get your wife or children to bring the snacks to you!)

- Avoid any regularity of exercise by: parking your car closest to work at the parking lot; never taking the stairs (always ride the elevator); using a power mower on the lawn or putting in colored rock to eliminate mowing entirely.

- Hire a gardener, painter, plumber, et cetera.

3. SMOKE HEAVILY, AND FOR MANY YEARS

- Everybody knows that there is at least twice as much heart disease in the group who competes here—with twice as many deaths. And don't forget the "help" you get in your project by the early development of many cancers (not just lung cancer), emphysema, hardening of the arteries of feet, legs, brain, et cetera.

4. DRINK ALCOHOLIC BEVERAGES

- Even "moderation" for the fellow who already has a little narrowing of the blood vessels that supply his heart increases his risk of heart failure and death significantly (by increasing workload of the heart without increasing the blood circulating to it).

5. DRIVE YOURSELF HARD

- Remember the goals and that there is "plenty of room at the top."

- Push, drive, fight all day long.

- When you come home, bring lots of work from the office.

- Never forget the work that must be done if you are going to become that junior (or senior) executive.

- Don't take time for recreation or vacations.

6. LIVE STRESSFULLY

- Emotional stress helps greatly to increase cholesterol in the blood stream. This cholesterol will be deposited easily and early in your blood vessels. Remember that the American soldiers under great stress and a high-fat—high-animal-fat—diet who died in combat during the Korean War were shown to have fantastic narrowing and hardening of their coronary arteries with cholesterol. (The U.S. Army did autopsies on the bodies of all these men they could recover from the combat zone.) The arteries of many 19-year-olds looked like the average 50-year-old male of the United States!

- Never take time for spiritual growth. Don't take your burdens to God or accept His promise to carry your yoke and make it light. If you did, your stresses would be reduced appreciably.

7. DRINK PLENTY OF COFFEE

- If you drink at least six cups a day, a very positive correlation has been shown (by Dr. Paul Ogelsby of Northwestern

University School of Medicine) to exist between coffee drinking and the development of heart disease.

• If you have a borderline disease already, the added caffeine will increase the irritability of your heart and help produce abnormal rhythm.

8. NEVER GET A PHYSICAL CHECKUP BY YOUR PHYSICIAN

• Early detection and care of your high blood pressure, diabetes, or hypothyroidism might result in your getting and keeping your cholesterol down.

• You might detect early (while treatable) the narrowing of your coronary arteries.

If you find yourself identifying with one or more of these behaviors, maybe now is the time to start thinking more seriously about what you can do to avoid heart disease.

What is Heart Disease?

Heart disease is not a single disease, but rather a multifaceted disease of various origins and types. The one which will be discussed in greatest detail here is coronary artery disease (CAD), also called atherosclerosis. This particular cardiovascular disease demands our attention because of the crucial role it plays in causing other degenerative disorders.

In order to take better care of the cardiovascular system, we need to understand its components and how they operate. The cardiovascular system consists of the heart, which maintains the flow of blood and the blood vessels which carry it. Blood circulates twice throughout the body every minute. Arter-

FIG. 6-1

DEATHS DUE TO CARDIOVASCULAR DISEASES BY MAJOR TYPE OF DISORDER
UNITED STATES: 1976
From National Center for Health Statistics. USPHS, DHEW

ies carry blood away from the heart, while veins carry blood back to the heart. Fig. 6-2 illustrates the flow of blood through the heart.

The primary function of the cardiovascular system is the transportation of oxygen, nutritive materials, and water to the cells, along with the transportation of carbon dioxide, urea, and other waste products to the proper organs for excretion.

The heart, which weighs about a half pound, and is about the size of a clenched fist, normally beats about 72 times per minute, or about 100,000 times per day. It's an amazing

FIG. 6–2

CORONARY CIRCULATION

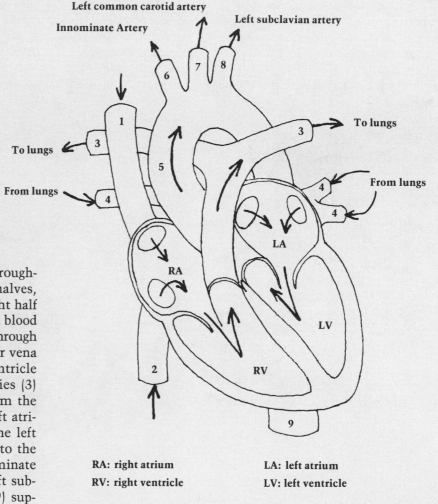

The heart muscle contracts and relaxes to pump blood through-out the circulatory system. The heart is divided into 2 halves, left and right; each half is divided into 2 cavities. The right half contains blood from the veins, the left, newly oxygenated blood from the lungs. Blood enters the right atrium of the heart through two large veins, the superior vena cava (1) and the inferior vena cava (2). It flows from the right atrium into the right ventricle and is pumped from there through the pulmonary arteries (3) to the lungs. In the lungs, the blood is oxygenated. From the lungs, it flows through the pulmonary veins (4) to the left atrium, and from the left atrium into the left ventricle. The left ventricle contracts, forcing the blood through the aorta to the body. Blood is carried to the upper body through the innominate artery (6), the left common carotid artery (7), and the left subclavian artery (8). The descending branch of the aorta (9) supplies the lower body.

RA: right atrium

RV: right ventricle

LA: left atrium

LV: left ventricle

organ. Try opening and closing your fist 72 times per minute, for a few minutes, and see how your hand feels.

The heart is composed of muscle tissue called the myocardium. The myocardium requires a continuous blood supply as do all muscles. However, instead of coming through the heart, the myocardium's blood supply is delivered through the coronary arteries which surround it. The three major coronary arteries are (1) the right coronary artery, (2) the left coronary artery, and (3) the circumflex branch of the left coronary artery (see Fig. 6–3). These are the arteries that are of primary concern when we talk about heart disease.

If the heart is so strong, why then does it eventually collapse? The etiology (the science or theory of the causes or origins of diseases) is very complex. There is no question that one of the primary causes of heart failure or heart attack is atherosclerosis.

FIG. 6–3

THE HEART AND THE CORONARY ARTERIES

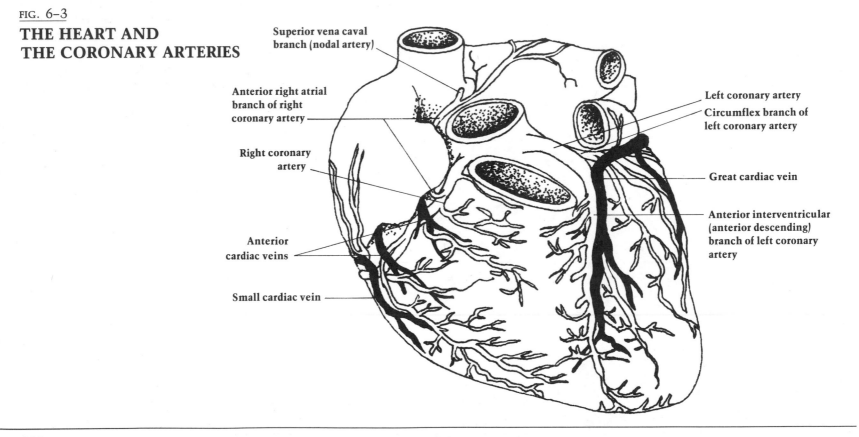

Superior vena caval branch (nodal artery)

Anterior right atrial branch of right coronary artery

Right coronary artery

Anterior cardiac veins

Small cardiac vein

Left coronary artery

Circumflex branch of left coronary artery

Great cardiac vein

Anterior interventricular (anterior descending) branch of left coronary artery

WHAT IS ATHEROSCLEROSIS?

Atherosclerosis is a degenerative disease which sets the stage for heart attacks and strokes. When sufficient deposits of soft fatty substances are made along the inside walls of the blood vessels, they begin to narrow, and the formation of atherosclerosis begins. When this occurs in the coronary arteries, the rate of blood flow and the amount of blood going to the heart muscle may be reduced to the point where a heart attack occurs. In some cases, the immediate trigger of the attack is a blood clot, or thrombus, which blocks an artery already narrowed by atherosclerosis. This kind of heart attack is called a coronary thrombus. A more transient inadequacy of blood supply to the heart may produce chest pains known as angina pectoris.[2]

Investigators are finding that atherosclerosis begins at a very early age in this country. Fatty streaks, for example, have been observed in the aortas of infants less than a year old.[3] During the Korean and Vietnam wars, many men in their early twenties were killed. In both of these wars, several studies were performed on the hearts of hundreds of these young soldiers killed in battle to see how widespread heart disease was among American soldiers.

One study reported in the Journal of The American Medical Association, involved 300 soldiers killed in Korea. The average age of these men was about 22 years. Of the autopsies performed on these soldiers, more than 50% had artery damage from plaques in the coronary arteries. A comparable group of Koreans, also killed in that war, showed virtually no evidence of this disease.[4]

In another study involving more than 100 American soldiers killed in South Vietnam, 50% of the autopsies showed normal coronary arteries, 45% had medium artery damage, and 5% had severe artery damage. The average age of the soldiers in South Vietnam was also about 22 years.[5]

Plaque is the substance which clogs or blocks the arteries. It consists of deposits of fibrin (clotting material), cholesterol, calcium, and cellular debris (cells which are either dead or in the process of dying due to lack of oxygen and nutrients caused by the formation of plaque).

Nathan Pritikin cites a study by C.J. Pepine on coronary heart disease which was discovered in asymptomatic men. "Pepine had observed that 30% of navy men dying of natural causes were under forty years of age and had no history of cardiovascular disease—yet this was the principal postmortem finding. He recruited forty-one navy and marine fliers, all under forty, and certified to be in excellent health by military diagnostic tests. His plan was to take these asymptomatic subjects and run angiograms on them every two years to monitor any developing coronary heart disease (An angiogram is the injection of a dye into an artery which is then X-rayed to show the shape of the artery or to determine if there is any blockage.) His baseline findings were unexpected: nineteen of the forty-one supposedly healthy men had advanced coronary heart disease; sixteen of them had two or three coronary arteries which were more than 50% blocked. Two years later, three of the subjects suffered heart attacks and four others were found to have worsened."[6]

The importance of these studies is twofold. They show, first, that heart disease may affect you at a very early age without any manifestation of symptoms; and second, that by the time physical exams discover the presence of heart disease, the disease may be considerably advanced.

What Causes a Heart Attack?

A heart attack is caused by a wide variety of factors. There is no *single* cause, even though we have a tendency to adhere to the idea of a single cause. How often have you heard someone say, "I can't understand why all of a sudden he had a heart attack. He was healthy and never sick a day in his life. What went wrong?"

By now I'm sure that you understand that most heart attacks and strokes are never really sudden. The formation of "yellow chicken fat" (plaque) may begin its destructive work many years before the actual heart attack. By the time most people reach their late forties or early fifties, if they're on a high-fat, high-cholesterol diet, smoking, obese, sedentary, and hypertensive, they're perfect candidates for a heart attack or stroke. Heredity also plays an important role.

A study completed a few years ago in Baltimore found that 30% to 40% of people with heart attacks complained of fatigue for weeks or months prior to their attacks. It is estimated that about one-third of all heart attacks are "silent," or minor and often not acknowledged.[7]

Whenever I lecture on heart disease, I inevitably hear about someone's grandmother who's lived to be 100 years old, smokes a package of cigarettes per day, eats lots of fat, and has never exercised a day in her life. Despite what we might like to believe, people who have lived to a ripe old age, but have disregarded the risk factors, are more the exception than the rule. There are no guarantees in life, but we can act to reduce some of the risks that lead to heart attack and stroke.

Let's examine some of the risk factors in more detail:

DIET

If you're on a high-fat, high-cholesterol diet, i.e., eating a lot of foods such as red meat, cream, butter, whole milk, and eggs, you are increasing your cholesterol and triglyceride levels. These eating habits represent one of the major risk factors in heart disease.

The following chart shows the results of a study done at the Cleveland Clinic in Cleveland, Ohio involving 723 young men with slight chest pain.[8]

FIG. 6–4

Cholesterol Level	% of Significant Artery Closure
Less than 200	20%
201–225	38%
226–250	48%
251–275	60%
276–300	77%
301–350	80%
More than 350	91%

As you can see, the cholesterol levels of the patients studied directly correlates with the percentage of significant artery closure. The higher the cholesterol level, the higher the percentage of blocked arteries.

When one or more of the coronary arteries becomes blocked, the danger of a heart attack increases. A practical suggestion to help keep your arteries clean, without oversimplifying a very complex problem, is: Look at your plate after you finish eating. If your plate is greasy and oily, your arteries are going to be greasy and oily, particularly if you're having one high-fat meal after another. This is how all that fatty substance begins to accumulate in your arteries. On the other hand, if your plate is clean, such as after you finish having a salad, you will help to keep your arteries clean and open. You don't need to get fanatical about this, however. If you go to the "Greasy Spoon" or "Ptomaine Harry's" once in a while, that's okay. It's having one high-fat meal after another, day in and day out, that can be harmful.

SMOKING

Everyone knows about the dangers of smoking, so I won't dwell on this point, except to say that if you smoke cigarettes, you are two to three times more likely to have a heart attack than non-smokers or former smokers.

EXERCISE

There's no longer any question about the value of exercise and its relationship to heart disease. Numerous studies have reinforced its importance. However, it's essential that it be the right type of exercise—aerobic exercise. As explained in Chapter 2, the pulse rate should be elevated 70% to 85% while exercising. Exercise not only helps to strengthen the heart muscle, but it also helps to lower blood pressure, cholesterol, triglycerides and in some cases relieves angina.

One other significant change which occurs with exercise is *collateral circulation*, which is the ingrowth of additional blood vessels. When a coronary artery supplying blood to a portion of the heart muscle is blocked, changes may occur in the coronary network that enable blood from other arteries to reach the affected area of the myocardium. Also, small collateral arteries may form to bypass the blocked or narrowed artery. Autopsies and some studies have verified this process.[9]

In a classic experiment, Dr. R.W. Eckstein used two groups of dogs: forty-four were experimental, and forty-six were controls. For both groups, subgroups were formed in which ligatures (thread or wire) of varying degrees of restriction were tied around the circumflex coronary artery in order to stimulate different degrees of coronary heart disease. The control groups were restricted to their cages; the experimental dogs exercised four times daily on a treadmill for a total of forty to fifty-six hours over a period of six to eight weeks. At the end of the experiment, the increase in collateral circulation of the exercised dogs was proportional to the degree of arterial constriction in the sedentary dogs. However, no increased collateral circulation occurred at all with mild constriction *unless* accompanied by exercise.[10]

Collateral circulation is one of the most important reasons for exercise, and one that I have always exphasized. If you've developed collateral circulation, it may be keeping you alive at this very moment, since most of us already have a certain amount of blockage in our arteries. If you haven't been exercising, now is the time to get started. It's never too late!

HYPERTENSION (HIGH BLOOD PRESSURE)

Hypertension, according to the American Heart Association, is one of the most insidious factors in heart attack and stroke, because it presents no characteristic symptoms and yet should be diagnosed and treated by a physician. Modern medicine has not yet identified the basic cause of hypertension. However, the condition can be controlled with a wide variety of drugs. It may not be the most desirable mode of treatment because of the innumerable side effects, but at the moment, drug therapy is the most effective approach. Needless to say, an attempt is made to discourage the use of drugs, unless they're absolutely essential. Anti-hypertensive medication, according to cardiologist George Sheehan, has many side effects, including decrease in water, salt, and potassium, and an increase in uric acid and sugar levels. However, its primary effect is on the central nervous system.

There are some individuals who have gradually been able to stop using their medication altogether. This, of course, has been done with a physician's guidance. (Prescribed medications of any kind should not be terminated abruptly without the knowledge and supervision of a physician.) On occasion,

I do come in contact with physicians who believe that a patient on anti-hypertensive medication, will always be on anti-hypertensive medication. This, of course, is sheer nonsense. Sweeping generalizations, such as these, do not apply to every patient. Many physicians have taken patients off medication altogether with the following recommendations:

• Start an aerobic exercise program (rope jumping, jogging, walking at a brisk pace, cycling, swimming, or any combination of these activities).

• Decrease salt to about two to three grams per day.

• Decrease fat intake.

• If overweight, decrease weight to your ideal weight through gradual, systematic undereating.

• Identify the sources of stress, tension, and anxiety in your life, and work on eliminating or reducing them as much as possible.

There is also another form of high blood pressure called idiopathic (of unknown origin) hypertension. Idiopathic hypertension cannot be directly attributed to stress, tension, kidney problems, or obesity.

If you're hypertensive, keep a close watch on your blood pressure, and have it checked on a regular basis. Many physicians recommend that the systolic (top number) blood pressure be no higher than 140 mm Hg (millimeters of mercury), and the diastolic (bottom number) blood pressure not exceed 90 mm Hg. However, most physicians consider 150/90 as borderline hypertension, while others feel that blood pressure is only abnormal if it is more than 160/95.

What is the Relationship Between Diabetes and Heart Disease?

The underlying cause of diabetes is one of the toughest problems facing medical researchers. For reasons not fully understood, individuals with diabetes are more susceptible to heart attack and stroke than their non-diabetic counterparts. At present, 250,000 new cases of diabetes are diagnosed annually in the U.S. Due to the overwhelming incidence of this disease, research into the prevention and cure of diabetes continues to be a priority.

In the past, it was thought that diabetes occurred only when the pancreas failed to produce enough insulin. In some instances, this is the case, because the cells in the pancreas which are involved with the production of insulin (islets of Langerhans), in some unknown way, often become damaged. In a number of diabetics, however, the pancreas appears to be perfectly normal.

At least in some cases then, the body may make the normal amount of insulin, but cannot use it effectively, or else needs a greater than normal amount. One of the areas that researchers are examining, is the relationship of fat to insulin. Some scientists are finding that an increase in fats produces a decrease in the efficiency of insulin.[11] Also, some studies have found that diabetics have higher levels of fat in their blood.[12]

Excessive consumption of simple sugars, such as white and brown sugar and syrups, have also been linked to diabetes.

Diabetes is a very complex degenerative disease. It is by no means one-dimensional. Basic factors associated with the onset of diabetes are:

AGE: 70% of diabetics are more than forty-five years old when diagnosed.

SEX: Women are 50% more likely to develop diabetes than men.

OBESITY: 85% of diabetics are overweight at the time of onset.

PREGNANCY: Women who have borne children weighing more than nine pounds at birth are prone to develop the disease later.[13]

Therefore, those who are most likely to have diabetes are relatives of diabetics, those who are overweight, and those who are at least forty-five years of age. But anyone, at any time, can develop diabetes.

In answer to the original question, the precise relationship between diabetes and heart disease is still under investigation, although diet is obviously a significant factor in both conditions.

What Are Some Other Risk Factors in Heart Disease?

BEHAVIOR CHARACTERISTICS

Are you a type A or type B personality?[14] In other words, are you impatient and hard-driving (type A) or relaxed and easy-going (type B)? Have you become a slave to time? How well do you cope with stress?

Studies have shown that individuals who are hard-driving, impatient, aggressive, and constantly aware of time are by far greater candidates for heart attacks than those who are generally relaxed and easy-going.

OBESITY

Obesity, as I've already indicated, is not only one of the risk factors of heart disease, but may also cause high blood pressure, varicose veins, poor blood supply to the lower extremities, and osteoarthritis. Obesity is also a serious complication in gallbladder disease and diabetes, and poses a problem for those with asthma, since excess weight is an added strain for the already overburdened heart and lungs.[15]

HEREDITY, AGE, SEX, AND RACE

These are additional risk factors. The following charts (Fig. 6–5 and 6–6) will help you to score your risk factors. The presence of more than one risk factor tends to multiply, not simply add to, the total risk.

Can Atherosclerosis Be Reversed or Arrested?

This is a very controversial question that has not yet been satisfactorily resolved. Studies by Lyons, involving 280 patients with histories of heart attacks appear to indicate that reversal may be possible.[16] Blankenhorn did another study involving 25 patients with femoral atherosclerosis. He used computer techniques to analyze the angiograms. Blankenhorn demonstrated regression in 9 of the 25 patients.[17]

Dr. Laurence Favrot, Associate Director of the Cardiac center, Sharp Hospital in San Diego, believes that an exercise and dietary program may not be adequate for everyone. "There are some patients that are too far along with coronary heart disease to cure," Dr. Favrot states. "Since we're dealing with a situation that is quite critical, it might be dangerous to proceed with purely an exercise and dietary program." He also points out that, "the medical management generally consists of: (1) decreasing the workload of the heart with medication; (2) dilators of the coronary arteries, usually in the form of nitrates; and (3) of course, a hygenic program of diet and exercise."[18]

More studies need to be done to reinforce the work of Dr. Blankenhorn and Dr. Lyons before any definitive conclusions can be drawn.

FIG. 6–5

SCORING YOUR RISK FACTORS

To determine your risk, complete the Risk Factor Score Form as follows:

1. For each risk factor, locate and circle the risk level that best describes you.

2. In the small box in the right-hand side of each risk level you circled, you'll find a numerical value in the far right-hand score column.

3. Follow this procedure and complete all ten risk factors.

4. Total the score column and enter your score in the box at the bottom entitled Total Risk Score.

5. See Profiling Your Risk of Attack (Fig. 6–6) to determine your own risk profile.

Risk Factor	Risk Level A well below average		Risk Level B below average		Risk Level C borderline		Risk Level D above average		Risk Level E dangerous level		Risk Level F urgent level		Score
Tobacco smoking	Never smoked	0	Quit smoking more than one year ago, or smoke cigar or pipe now	1	Quite smoking less than one year ago or now smoke 10 cig. day max.	2	20 cigarettes per day	4	30 cigarettes per day	6	40 or more cigarettes per day	8	
Behavior Characteristics	Always easy going and calm	1	Easy going and calm most of the time	2	Frequently impatient and clock-watching	3	Persistently driving for advancement in work and play	4	Overwhelming ambition, slavish to time & deadlines	6	Hard-driving, hard-charging, can never relax	8	
Age	10–20 years	0	21–30 years	1	31–40 years	2	41–50 years		51–60 years		61 years & up	5	
Gender	Female under 40	0	Female 40–50	1	Female over 50	2	Male	3	Stocky male	4	Bald, stocky male	5	
Family History (parents, grandparents, brothers & sisters only)	No known history of heart disease	1	One relative with heart disease over age 60	2	Two relatives with heart disease over age 60	3	One relative with heart disease under age 60	4	Two relatives with heart disease under age 60	6	Three relatives with heart disease under age 60	7	
Weight	More than 5 lbs. below standard weight	0	–5 lbs. to + 5 lbs. of standard weight	1	6–20 lbs. overweight	3	21–35 lbs. overweight	3	36–50 lbs. overweight	5	51 + lbs. overweight	7	
Exercise (Subtract 1 point if you participate in regular aerobic exercise)	Intensive occupational & recreational exertion	1	Moderate occupational & recreational exertion	2	Sedentary work & intense recreational exertion	3	Sedentary work and moderate recreational exertion	4	Sedentary work and light recreational exertion	5	Sedentary work with no exercise	6	
Diabetes (parents, grandparents, brothers	No known family history	1	One relative with diabetes	2	Two relatives with diabetes	3	Diabetes in yourself beginning after age 60	4	Diabetes in yourself beginning between 20 & 60	6	Diabetes in yourself beginning before age 20	8	
Cholesterol (mg/100 ml) If you do not know your level, use 231–255	Below 180	1	180–205	2	206–230	3	231–255	4	256–280	6	281 or more	8	
Blood Pressure (Upper Reading) If you do not know your BP, use 140	Less than 120	1	130 max.	2	140 max.	3	160 max.	4	180 max.	6	200 & over	8	

Total Risk Score

FIG. 6–6

PROFILING YOUR RISK OF HEART ATTACK

STEP 1:
Use the following table to profile your risk of heart attack:

If your risk score is between:	Your risk is:	You're encouraged to take the following action:
6–15	Well below average	Keep up the good work. You're within acceptable limits.
16–21	High end of acceptable	Note any risk factors that fall into Levels D, E & F. Take action to modify them. Consult your physician before beginning your risk factor modification program.
22–29	Borderline	Your risk factors deserve attention. You should consult your physician for a cardiovascular checkup to determine the current status of your heart and to develop a program to promptly lower those risks that fell into levels D, E, & F. (See Step 2 below)
30–39	Above average	IMMEDIATE ATTENTION ADVISED. Your risk factors must be lowered to reduce your risk of heart attack or stroke! Contact your physician for a complete cardiovascular checkup. Through new procedures, your physician can determine the status of your heart and predict your susceptibility to heart attack. Your physician will discuss your risk factors and help you lower your risk. Act now . . . follow directions outlined in Step 2 below.
40–50	High	
above 51	Very high	

Note: The scores and relative risks are based on *statistical data*. The profile cannot constitute a diagnosis or a health guarantee, because the significance of risk factors varies with individuals. This program simply offers you a method to evaluate your statistical chances of suffering a heart attack or stroke.

STEP 2

Acceptable Range:

If your Total Risk Score fell between 6 and 21, complete the following:

Although your Total Risk Score indicated a relatively low risk, there is significance to having *two or more* above-average risk factors.

Return to the Risk Factor Score form and count the number of risk levels (other than age and gender) you circled in risk levels D, E and F. Count circles only, not numerical values in the boxes.

If you count two or more risk levels, discuss those risk factors with your physician; enlist his or her aid in developing a modification program.

Note: Risk factor profiling can identify upwards of 70% of individuals who will experience a heart attack or stroke. The remaining 30% of the heart attack or stroke victims exhibit below average risk factors. Hence, absence of high risk factors does not exclude you from the possibility of having a cardiovascular incident.

You should commence a cardiovascular health improvement plan to further reduce your risk. Before undertaking such a program, consult your physician regarding a treadmill exercise test. This test provides the information needed to determine the current condition of your heart and to prescribe safe levels of exercise.

Borderline and Above:

If your Total Risk Score was 22 or above, you owe it to yourself and your family to take positive action. Remember, reduction of your risk factors can stave off the development of heart disease and result in a longer and healthier life.

It is important that before you begin your risk factor reduction program you see your physician for a treadmill exercise test to determine the current condition of your heart. This test is especially important if you have high risk factors, even though you may show no outward symptoms or may have a normal resting electrocardiogram.

By determining the current condition of your heart, your physician will have the information needed to safely and accurately prescribe the type of relative urgency of your cardiovascular health improvement program.

Under your physician's guidance, you can safely modify your risk factors, improve your physical condition and be on your way to a healthier, happier life.

Don't play ostrich with your heart. Take this next and important step . . . today.

Regardless of your risk profile, *under no circumstances* should you engage in a physical fitness program which entails a greater level of exertion than you normally undertake without first consulting your physician.

FIG. 6–7

WHAT YOU SHOULD KNOW ABOUT HEART ATTACK

An estimated 4,190,000 have coronary heart disease. 646,073 died of heart attack in 1976—350,000 before they reached the hospital. Many thousands of these might have been saved if the victims had heeded the signals.

Delay spells danger. When you suffer a heart attack, minutes—especially the first few minutes—count.

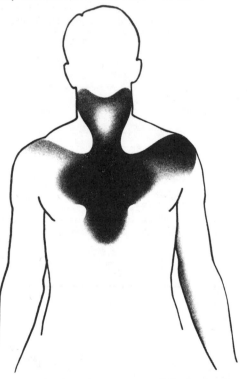

INTENSITY AND LOCATION OF PAIN

KNOW THE SIGNALS

Signals vary . . . but the usual warnings of heart attack are:

• Uncomfortable pressure, fullness, squeezing or pain in the center of the chest for more than two minutes.

• Pain may spread to the shoulders, neck or arms.

• Severe pain, dizziness, fainting, sweating, nausea or shortness of breath may also occur.

• These signals are not always present. Sometimes they subside and then return.

EMERGENCY ACTION

If you are having typical chest discomfort which lasts for two minutes or more, call the local emergency rescue service immediately. If you can get to a hospital faster by car, have someone drive you. Find out which hospitals have 24-hour emergency cardiac care and discuss with your doctor the possible choices. Plan in advance the route that's best from where you live and work. Keep a list of emergency rescue service numbers next to your telephone and in a prominent place in your pocket, wallet or purse.

BE A HEART SAVER

If you are with someone who is having the signals, and if they last for two minutes or longer, act at once.

Expect a "denial." It is normal to deny the possibility of anything as serious as a heart attack—but insist on taking prompt action.

You can start today to reduce the risk factors over which you have control. An excellent place to begin is with the Sensible Diet. By eating properly you automatically reduce many of the risk factors. Risk factors which neither you nor your doctor can control—age, sex and heredity—obviously can't be modified. But there is still a great deal you can do. How much is up to you. You're in control of your body, so you decide how you want it to function. You're in control of your emotions, so you decide how you want them to be expressed. You're in control of your mind, so you decide whether you will allow it to function within a positive or negative framework. If it's positive, you're on the right track, otherwise you've got some work to do.

You can develop your own "lean machine." Do it on your own or with your friends and family. It's never too late. I know a beautiful lady in Los Angeles by the name of Eula Weaver who started exercising when she was in her eighties. She's now ninety-two years old, jogs one-and-a-half miles and cycles fifteen miles every day. She has competed in the Senior Olympics, won several gold medals, and on top of that has a boyfriend she's crazy about. This is what life is all about. Most men are considered middle-aged by the time they reach twenty-seven. That's why you're better off being ninety-two years *young*, rather than twenty-seven years *old*.

Enjoy life and love life since our time on this earth is limited. Count your blessings, be thankful for what you have, and always keep moving—but in the right direction.

Notes

1. STRETCHING

1. Hans Kraus, *Clinical Treatment of Back and Neck Pain* (New York: McGraw-Hill, 1970).

2. PULSE-RATED EXERCISE

1. Laurence Morehouse and Leonard Gross, *Total Fitness in 30 Minutes a Week* (New York: Simon and Schuster, 1976), p. 135.

3. ROPE JUMPING

1. J. Joyce, A. DeMaria, J. Giddeno et al., "Exercise Induced Decreases in Platelet Aggregation: Comparison of Normals and Coronary Patients Showing Similar Physical Activity Related Effects," *American Journal of Cardiology* 41 (1978): 432.

2. Kaare Rodahl in Curtis Mitchell, *The Perfect Exercise: The Hop, Skip and Jump Way to Health* (New York: Simon and Schuster, 1976), pp. 20–21.

3. *Ibid.*, p. 21.

4. John A. Baker, "Comparison of Rope Skipping and Jogging as Methods of Improving Cardiovascular Efficiency of College Men," *The Research Quarterly* (American Association for Health, Physical Education, and Recreation, May 1968): 240–43.

5. Kenneth H. Cooper, *The New Aerobics* (New York: Evans and Co., Inc., 1970).

6. From "The Cause and Cure of Side Stitch," *Executive Fitness Newsletter* (Emmaus, Pa., Sept. 8, 1973).

7. Robert Kerlan, M.D. and Frank Jobe, M.D., National Athletic Health Institute Booklet, Los Angeles, 1977, p. 46.

8. Consumer Reports, eds. *The Medicine Show* (New York: Pantheon Books, 1974), pp. 224–225.

9. Morehouse and Gross, *Total Fitness in 30 Minutes a Week*, pp. 42–43.

10. *Guinness Book of Word Records*, 1977.

4. THE SENSIBLE DIET

1. William Glasser, M.D., *Positive Addiction* (New York: Harper & Row, 1976)

2. Paavo Airola, Ph.D.,M.D., *How to Get Well* (Phoenix: Health Plus, 1974)

3. Nathan Pritikin et al., *Live Longer Now* (New York: Grosset and Dunlap, 1974), p. 59.

4. Thomas Jukes, "The Simple Truth about Sugar," *Runners World* (December 1978): 57.

5. I.L. Shannon et al., "Honey: Sugar Content and Cariogenicity," *ASDC Journal of Dentistry for Children* 46 (1979): 29.

6. W.B. Kannel et al., "Vascular Disease of the Brain, Epidemilogic Aspects: Framingham Study," *American Journal of Public Health*, 55 (1965): 1355.

7. F.R. Lemon and R.T. Walden, "Death from Respiratory System Disease Among Seventh-Day Adventist Men," *Journal of the American Medical Association* 198 (1966): 117.

8. Gordon H. Theilen, DVM et al., "Leukemia in Animals and Man," *California Medicine* 108 (January 1968): 14–19.

9. Jean Snyder, "About the Meat You Are Buying," *Today's Health* (December 1971): 39.

10. Stoy Proctor, *Unmeat: The Case for Vegetarianism* (Nashville, Tennessee: Southern Publishing Association, 1973): 29.

11. "Number of Carcasses Retained for Various Diseases and Conditions but Passed for Food after Removal of Affected Parts," (Washington, D.C.: Department of Agriculture Report, Fiscal Year 1972): p. 6.

12. Corinne H. Robinson, *Basic Nutrition and Diet Therapy* (New York: Macmillan Co., 1970), pp. 196–7.

13. Robin Hur, *Food Reform: Our Desperate Need* (Austin, Texas: Heidelberg Publishers, 1975), p. 124.

14. R. Hedman, "The Available Glycogen in Man and the Connection between Rate of Oxygen Intake and Carbohydrate Usage," *Acta Physiology Scandinavia* 40 (1957): 305–309.

15. Per-Olof Astrand, "Something Old and Something New. . . . Very New," *Nutrition Today* (1968), p. 9.

16. M. Friedman et al., "The Effect of Unsaturated Fats Upon Lipemia and Conjunctival Circulation," *JAMA*, 193 (1965): 882.

17. M. Bierenbaum et al., "The Five Year Experience of Modified Fat Diets on Younger Men with Coronary Heart Disease," *Circulation* 42 (1970): 943.

18. Samuel Bellet, "Response of Free Fatty Acids to Coffee and Caffeine," *Metabolism* 17 (1968): 702–708.

19. D.W. Edington and V.R. Edgerton, *The Biology of Physical Activity* (Boston: Houghton Mifflin Co., 1976), p. 312.

20. M. Hamilton and E. Whitney, *Nutrition Concepts and Controversies* (New York: West Publishing Co.), p. 381.

21. From a conversation with Dr. Cleaves Bennett, Medical Director of the Longevity Center (Santa Monica, California, 1979).

22. Nathan Pritikin, J. Leonard and J. Hofer, *Live Longer Now*, p. 146.

23. A. Keys, "Coronary Heart Disease in Seven Countries," *Circulation* 41, Supp. 1 (1970).

24. Nathan Pritikin and Patrick M. McGrady, Jr., *The Pritikin Program for Diet and Exercise* (New York: Grosset and Dunlap, 1979), p. 364.

25. C.C. Welch, "Cinecoronary Arteriography in Young Men," *Circulation* 62 (1970): 625.

26. John Yiamouyiannis, M.D., "Fluoridation and Cancer," *Cancer Control Journal* 5 (1978): 38–41.

27. Dean Burk, M.D., "Fluoridation and Cancer, Age-Dependence of Cancer Mortality Related to Artificial Fluoridation," *Ibid.*, p. 27.

28. Albert Burgstahler, Ph.D., "Brief Report on Water Fluoridation," *Ibid.*, pp. 49–53.

29. Hamilton and Whitney, *Nutrition Concepts and Controversies* pp. 295–296.

30. J.M. Coon, "Natural Food Toxicants: A Perspective," *Nutrition Review* (1976): 538.

31. R.J. Hickey and R.G. Clelland, "Hazardous Food Additives: Nitrite and Saliva?" *New England Journal of Medicine* 298 (1978): 1036.

32. Julie Waltz, "Controlling Eating Environments," *Food Habit Management* (Seattle: Northwest Learning Associates, Inc., 1978), pp. 267–269.

5. VITAMINS

1. Paavo Airola, *Are You Confused?* (Phoenix: Health Plus Publishers, 1971), p. 49.

2. "Some Facts and Myths of Vitamins," *FDA Consumer* (U.S. Dept. of Health, Education and Welfare, Publication No. 79–2117, 1979).

3. Expert Panel on Food Safety and Nutrition, Committee on Public Information, Institute of Food Technologists, "Vitamin E," *Contemporary Nutrition*, 2 (November 1977).

4. A.L. Tappel, "Vitamin E," *Nutrition Today* (July/August 1973): 4–12.

5. H.H. Draper, J.G. Bergan, M. Chiu, A.S. Csallany, and A.V. Boaro, "A Further Study of the Specificity of the Vitamin E Requirement for Reproduction," *Journal of Nutrition*, 84 (1964): 395–400.

6. HEART DISEASE AND ITS PREVENTION

1. Richard T. Walden, M.D., F.A.C.P., "How to Die Younger," Health Media Services (Loma Linda, California, 1977).

2. "Update: Physical Activity and Coronary Heart Disease," *Physical Fitness Research Digest* Series 9, No. 2, April 1979.

3. R.L. Holman et al., "The Natural History of Atherosclerosis: The Early Aortic Lesions as Seen in New Orleans in the Middle of the 20th Century," *American Journal of Pathology* 34 (1958): 209–234.

4. W.F. Enos et al., "Pathogenesis of Coronary Disease in American Soldiers Killed in Korea," *Journal of the American Medical Association*, (July 16, 1955).

5. J.J. McNamara et al., "Coronary Artery Disease in Vietnam Casualties," *Journal of the American Medical Association* 216 (May 17, 1971): 1185–87.

6. Pritikin and McGrady, *The Pritikin Program for Diet and Exercise*, p. 365.

7. Irving M. Levitas, M.D., "Stress Testing: New Indications, New Techniques," *Diagnosis* (May/June, 1979).

8. C.C. Welch, "Cinecoronary Arteriography in Young Men," *Circulation* 62 (1970): 625.

9. "Update: Exercise and Some Coronary Risk Factors," *Physical Fitness Research Digest* Series 9, No. 3 (July 1979).

10. R.W. Eckstein, "Effects of Exercise and Coronary Heart Narrowing on Coronary Collateral Circulation," *Circulation Research* 5 (1957): 230.

11. V. Buber, "Improvement of Oral Glucose Tolerance by Acute Drug-Induced Lowering of Plasma-Free Fatty Acids," *Schweiz Med. Wschr.* 98 (1968): 711–12.

12. J.D. Bagdale, "Diabetic Lipemia," *New England Journal of Medicine* 276 (1967): 427–433.

13. Provided by the American Diabetes Association, Southern California Affiliate, Inc. (1975).

14. Meyer Friedman, *Type A Behavior and Your Heart* (New York: Knopf Publishers, 1974).

15. C. Seltzer and F.J. Stare, "Obesity," *Medical Insight* (July/August 1973): 12.

16. T.P. Lyons et al., "Lipoproteins and Diet in Coronary Heart Disease," *California Medicine* 84 (1956): 325.

17. D.H. Blankenhorn et al., "The Rate of Atherosclerosis Change during Treatment of Hyperlipoproteinemia," *Circulation* 57 (1978): 255–261.

18. Laurence Favrot, M.D., "Progression of Coronary Disease After Bypass Surgery: Can it Be Modified?" 3rd Annual Conference of the Pritikin Research Foundation (Santa Monica, California, 1979).

Bibliography

Airola, Paavo, Ph.D., M.D., *How to Get Well.* Phoenix: Health Plus, 1974.

Anderson, Bob, *Stretching.* Englewood, Colorado, 1975.

Astrand, Per-Olof, "Something Old and Something New . . . Very New." *Nutrition Today*, 1968, p. 9.

Astrand, Per-Olof, M.D. and Rodahl, Kaare, M.D., *Textbook of Work Physiology: Physiological Bases of Exercise.* New York: McGraw-Hill Book Company, 1977.

Bagdale, J.D. "Diabetic Lipemia." *New England Journal of Medicine* 276:427–433, 1967.

Baker, John A. "Comparison of Rope Skipping and Jogging as Methods of Improving Cardiovascular Efficiency of College Men." *Research Quarterly* (American Association for Health, Physical Education and Recreation, Washington, D.C.), May, 1968.

Bellet, S. "Response of Free Fatty Acids to Coffee and Caffeine." *Metabolism*, 17:702–708, 1968.

Blankenhorn, D.H., et al., "The Rate of Atherosclerosis Change During Treatment of Hyperlipoproteinemia." *Circulation* 57:355–361, 1978.

Cooper, Kenneth H. *The New Aerobics.* New York: Evans and Co., Inc., 1970.

Eckstein, R.W. "Effects of Exercise and Coronary Artery Narrowing on Coronary Collateral Circulation." *Circulation Research* Vol. 5, 1957, p. 230.

Edington, D.W.; Edgerton, V.R. *The Biology of Physical Activity.* Boston: Houghton Mifflin Co., 1976.

Enos, W.F. et al. "Pathogenesis of Coronary Disease in American Soldiers Killed in Korea." *JAMA*, July 16, 1955.

Falls, H.B.; Wallis, E.L.; Logan, G.A. *Foundations of Conditioning*, New York: Academic Press, Inc., 1970.

Filson, Sidney; Jessup, Claudie. *Jump into Shape.* New York: Franklin Watts, Inc., 1978.

Friedman, M., et al. "The Effect of Unsaturated Fats Upon Lipemia and Conjunctival Circulation." *JAMA* 193:882, 1965.

Glasser, William, M.D. *Positive Addiction.* Harper & Row, New York, 1976.

Guthrie, Helen Andrews. *Introductory Nutrition.* St. Louis: C.V. Mosby Co., 1971.

Hamilton, M.; Whitney E. *Nutrition Concepts and Controversies.* New York: West Publishing Co., 1979.

Hedman, R. "The Available Glycogen in Man and the Connection Between Rate of Oxygen Intake and Carbohydrate Usage." *Acta Physiol. Scand.* Vol. 40, 1957, pp. 305–309.

Holman, R.L., et al. "The Natural History of Atherosclerosis: The Early Aortic Lesions as Seen in New Orleans in the Middle of the 20th Century." *American Journal of Pathology* 34:209–234, 1958.

Hur, Robin. *Food Reform: Our Desperate Need.* Austin, Texas: Heidelberg Publishers, 1975, p. 124.

Joye, J.; Demaria, A.; Giddeno, Jr.; et al. "Exercise Induced Decreases in Platelet Aggregation: Comparison of Normals and Coronary Patients Showing Similar Physical Activity Related Effects." *American Journal of Cardiology* 41:432, 1978.

Keys, A. "Coronary Heart Disease in Seven Countries." *Circulation* 41, Suppl. 1, 1970.

Levitas, Irving M. "Stress Testing: New Indications, New Techniques." *Diagnosis*, May/June, 1979.

Lyons, T.P., et al. "Lipoproteins and Diet in Coronary Heart Disease." *California Medicine* 84:325, 1956.

McNamara, J.J., et al. "Coronary Artery Disease in Viet Nam Casualties." *JAMA*, May 17, 1971.

Mitchell, Curtis. *The Perfect Exercise: The Hop, Skip and Jump Way to Health.* New York: Simon and Schuster, 1976.

Morehouse, Laurence E., and Leonard Gross. *Total Fitness in 30 Minutes a Week.* New York: Simon and Schuster, 1975.

Page, Irvine H., et al. "Prediction of Coronary Heart Disease Based on Clinical Suspicion, Age, Total Cholesterol, and Triglyceride." *Circulation* 42, October, 1970.

Parrett, Owen S. *Diseases of Food Animals.* Washington, D.C.: Review and Herald Publishing Association, 1974, p. 4.

Pritikin, Nathan; Leonard, J.; Hofer, J. *Live Longer Now.* New York: Grosset and Dunlap, 1974.

Pritikin, Nathan and McGrady, Patrick M., Jr. *The Pritikin Program for Diet and Exercise*. New York: Grosset and Dunlap, 1979.

Robinson, Corinne H. *Basic Nutrition and Diet Therapy*. New York: Macmillan Co., 1970.

"Rope Skipping, Dancing, Walking, and Golf-Pack Carrying." *Physical Fitness Research Digest* Series 7, No. 4, October, 1977.

Seltzer, Carl C., Ph.D.; Stare, Frederick J., M.D. "Obesity." *Medical Insight*, July-August, 1973.

Shannon, I.L.; Edmonds, E.J.; Madsen, K.O. "Honey: Sugar Content and Cariogenicity." *ASDC. Journal of Dentistry for Children* 46:29, 1979.

Smith, Paul. *Rope Skipping: Rhythms, Routines and Rhymes*. Freeport, Educational Activities, Inc., 1969.

Snyder, Jean. "About the Meat You Are Buying." *Today's Health*, December, 1971, p. 29.

"Update: Exercise and Some Coronary Risk Factors." *Physical Fitness Research Digest* Series 9, No. 3, July, 1979.

"Update: Physical Activity and Coronary Heart Disease." *Physical Fitness Research Digest* Series 9, No. 2, April, 1979.

Waltz, Julie. *Food Habit Management*. Seattle: Northwest Learning Associates, Inc., 1978.

Glossary

Abductors—Muscles that are involved with movement away from the central axis of the body.

Abscess—A localized collection of pus surrounded by inflamed tissue.

Adductors—Muscles that are involved with movement toward the central axis of the body.

Aerobic Exercise—Exercise that requires an increase in oxygen intake over a period of time, including any activity that involves rhythmic motion of the large muscles such as rope jumping, jogging, cycling, swimming, etc.

Angiogram—Injection of a dye (radiopaque material) into blood vessels which are then x-rayed to determine if there is any blockage or restriction in blood flow.

Angina Pectoris—Pain in the heart region caused by lack of oxygen.

Anemia—A condition in which there is a reduced number of red blood cells or red blood cells with a reduced amount of hemoglobin. **Nutritional anemia** is a condition which results from a deficiency of certain essential nutrients in the diet such as iron, vitamins, and protein. **Pernicious anemia** is a genetic inability of the body to absorb vitamin B_{12}. This in turn affects the production of red blood cells, resulting in low levels of hemoglobin, as well as degeneration of the peripheral nerves.

Antibiotic—A soluble substance derived from a mold or bacteria that inhibits the growth of other microorganisms.

Anti-hypertensive Medication—Prescribed medication to lower high blood pressure.

Antioxidant—A compound that protects other compounds from oxygen by itself reacting with oxygen. Antioxidants retard the oxidation of unsaturated fats and oils, colorings and flavorings. Oxidation leads to loss of color, flavor changes and rancidity.

Aorta—The main artery of the body, carrying blood from the left ventricle of the heart to all branch arteries and organs except the lungs.

Appendicitis—Inflammation of the appendix.

Arteriosclerosis—Abnormal thickening and hardening of the arteries.

Artery—A vessel which carries blood away from the heart.

Arterial Constriction—The narrowing of the lumen (hollow cavity) of an artery.

Ascorbic Acid—The synthetic form of vitamin C.

Asymptomatic—Without symptoms, or producing no symptoms.

Atherosclerosis—An extreme form of arteriosclerosis in which fat, cholesterol crystals, fibrin, and dead cells form in the inner linings of the arteries and restrict circulation.

Atrioventricular—Relating to both the atria and the ventricles of the heart.

Atrium—The upper cavity of each half of the heart, which acts as a receiving chamber.

Atrophy—Degeneration or decrease in the size of an organ or cellular tissue.

Biotin—One of the B vitamins.

Blood Pressure—The pressure within the arteries pushing outward. **Systolic Pressure** is the pressure within the arteries upon ventricular contraction. **Diastolic pressure** is the pressure within the arteries upon ventricular relaxation.

Bradycardia—A decreased heart rate that is less than 60 beats per minute.

Brucellosis—An infectious disease characterized by fever, sweating, weakness, pains, and aches, sometimes becoming chronic and producing long lasting disability. It is ordinarily transmitted from animals.

Caffeine—A stimulant to the central nervous system, found mainly in tea, coffee, and cola drinks.

Calorie—The heat energy required to raise the temperature of 1 gram of water 1°C. (Also see kilocalorie.)

Capillaries—Tiny blood vessels that connect the smallest arteries and veins. Their walls are semipermeable, allowing exchange of substances between blood and tissue fluids.

Carbon Dioxide—A colorless, odorless gas that is formed when carbon combines with oxygen. It leaves the body chiefly when air is exhaled from the lungs.

Carbohydrate—An energy-yielding nutrient that consists of carbon, hydrogen, and oxygen, and is generally identified with starches and sugars.

Carcinogen—Cancer-causing substance.

Cardiovascular—Relating to the circulatory system, specifically the heart and blood vessels.

Cardiovascular Conditioning—Exercise which places emphasis on conditioning the heart and the blood vessels.

Caries—Decayed teeth.

Cariogenic—Producing tooth decay.

Carotid Artery—One of the large arteries on each side of the neck which supplies the external and internal tissues of the head and neck with blood.

Cartilage—A tough, firm connective tissue found in the joints. There are three kinds of cartilage: hyaline, elastic, and fibrocartilage.

Cellular Debris—Dead cells or cells which are in the process of dying.

Chelating Agents—Substances in foods that trap trace amounts of metal atoms that would otherwise cause food to discolor or go rancid.

Cholesterol—A fatlike substance manufactured primarily by the body, but also found in animal fats such as eggs, organ meats, and shellfish. **Serum Cholesterol** is the watery part of the blood which separates from the clot when blood coagulates.

Circumflex—One of the principle coronary arteries branching off the left coronary artery.

Cobalamin—Vitamin B_{12}.

Colitis—Inflammation of the colon.

Collateral Circulation—The ingrowth of additional blood vessels.

Colon—Portion of the large intestine between the cecum (where the large intestine begins) and the rectum.

Coma—A state of deep and prolonged unconsciousness often caused by injury or disease.

Coronary—Relating to either of two arteries branching from the aorta and supplying blood directly to the heart tissues.

Coronary Artery Disease—An abnormality in the vessels that supply blood to the heart.

Coronary Thrombosis—The formation of a clot in a branch of either of the coronary arteries, resulting in obstruction of that artery.

Dehydration—Deprivation of water or the reduction of water content.

Diabetes—A metabolic disease characterized by an inadequate supply of effective insulin, which renders a person unable to regulate blood glucose level normally. **Diabetic Coma** is a condition that results when sugar cannot be utilized and fat is called upon to supply the body's need for energy. When the limit to the amount of fat that the body can burn is reached, ketone bodies accumulate faster than the body can eliminate them, resulting in ketosis.

Diastolic (See Blood Pressure).

Distillation—A process of producing water by heating it into vapor and then allowing it to condense into liquid again. The process removes virtually all of the solids, minerals, and trace elements.

Diuretic—An agent or medication that causes increased water excretion.

Diverticulitis—Inflammation of the diverticulum, especially of the small pockets in the wall of the colon that fill with stagnant fecal material and become inflamed.

Diverticulum—A pouch or sac opening from a tubular or saccular organ such as the colon or bladder.

Dysfunction—Impaired functioning.

Edema—Swelling of a part of or the entire body caused by an accumulation of water.

Emulsifier—A surface-active agent, often used in foods to keep oil and water mixed together.

Enriched—Refers to a process by which the nutrients thiamin, riboflavin, niacin, and iron are added to refined grains and grain products at levels specified by law.

Epidemiology—A branch of medicine that investigates the causes and control of epidemics.

Epithelioma—A malignant tumor of epithelial cells, particularly of the skin, mouth, and larynx.

Etiology—The science or theory of the causes or origins of diseases.

Excretion—Elimination.

Fatty Acid—One of a class of compounds which are the building blocks of fats.

Fiber—The part of plant food which passes through the small intestine, not hydrolized (broken down) by the endogenous secretions, and on into the large intestine virtually unchanged.

Fibrin—An elastic, threadlike protein formed from fibrinogen. It's the principal protein material in a blood clot.

Flavor Enhancers—Food additives that have little or no flavor of their own, but accentuate the natural flavor of foods.

Fluoride—A compound of fluorine and one or more elements. It can be obtained in drinking water at a concentration of 1 ppm. It is recommended as an important health measure to protect children's teeth from decay and for the prevention of osteoporosis. Its use in drinking water is a controversial issue, as opponents claim it is cancer-causing.

Fluorine—A very active chemical element of the halogen family (chlorine, bromine, and iodine); a corrosive greenish-yellow gas.

Fortified—The addition of nutrients to foods, such as iron to breakfast cereals, vitamins A and D to milk, and iodine to salt.

Fructose—A monosaccharide sometimes referred to as fruit sugar, but also found in honey.

Gallstone—A solid mass in the gallbladder or a bile duct, composed chiefly of cholesterol crystals.

Glucose—A monosaccharide that is the simplest form of sugar.

Gluteal muscles—The muscles of the buttocks.

Gout—A metabolic disorder involving abnormal purine metabolism. Purines (nitrogen containing compounds) are normally converted to uric acid and eliminated in the urine. However, in gout, elevated uric acid levels are deposited as an insoluble salt in the joints, and usually manifested as attacks of arthritis.

Hamstrings—The muscles in the back of the thighs.

Heart Rate—The number of times the heart beats per minute.

Hemoglobin—The iron-containing protein of the red blood cells that combine with oxygen.

Hemorrhoids—A painful swelling or tumor of a vein in the anal or rectal region, caused by excessive venous pressure. Also known as *piles*.

Hepatitis (infectious)—Inflammation of the liver caused by a virus. Condition may be inapparent, mild, severe, and occasionally fatal. The disease is commonly seen in epidemics and transmission is by the fecal-oral route.

Hiatus Hernia—A protrusion of the upper part of the stomach through the diaphragm and into the upper chest cavity.

High Blood Pressure (See Hypertension).

Hormone—A chemical messenger. Hormones are secreted by a variety of endocrine glands in the body. Each affects a specific tissue or organ and elicits a specific response.

Hydrogenation—The "artificial hardening" of unsaturated fat or the process of adding hydrogen to unsaturated fat to make it more solid and to improve its storage life.

Hyperlipidemia—An abnormally high level of total fats in the blood.

Hypertension—Persistently high arterial blood pressure. **Idiopathic hypertension** is high blood pressure of unknown cause.

Hyperuricemia—A high level of uric acid in the blood.

Hypoglycemia—A condition characterized by an abnormally

low level of sugar in the blood (below about 60 or 70 mg per 100 ml).

Iodine—A "trace element," i.e., one essential to life in small quantities. It is extracted from seaweed, and used medically as an antiseptic and internally in thyroid disease. Iodine is a part of thyroxin, which is responsible for the basal metabolic rate.

Insulin—A hormone secreted by the pancreas and responsible for aiding the transport of glucose across cell membranes. **Insulin reaction** (too little sugar in the blood) is a disorder that occurs when the insulin level becomes upset, and the blood sugar level falls below the normal level.

Intercostal Muscles—The muscles located between the ribs.

Iron—An essential trace element. Most of the iron in the body is a component of the proteins hemoglobin and myoglobin, both of which carry oxygen and release it.

Ischemia—A deficit in oxygen availability, due to blockage of a blood vessel.

Islets of Langerhans—Endocrine glands of the pancreas which secrete the hormone insulin.

Ketosis—Condition resulting from the accumulation of ketones (acetone bodies) as a result of incomplete oxidation of fatty acids.

Kilocalorie (*k* cal)—The heat energy required to raise the temperature of 1 kg (1000 g) of water 1°C; also called *calorie*.

Kwashiorkor—A protein deficiency disease that occurs primarily among children between the ages of 2 and 5 years when they are weaned from mother's milk to a diet of starchy cereal pastes practically devoid of protein.

Legume—A plant of the bean and pea family. The seeds are rich in high-quality protein as compared with that of most other plant foods.

Leukemia—A disease of the blood-forming tissues, characterized by an abnormal and persistent increase in the number of white blood cells.

Ligament—Connective tissue attaching bone to bone.

Ligature—A thread or wire tied tightly around a blood vessel or other structure in order to constrict it.

Lipids—Broad term for fats and fat-like substances characterized by the presence of one or more fatty acids. Lipids include fats, cholesterol, lecithins, phospholipids, and similar substances.

Lipoprotein—A cluster of lipids surrounded by protein; serves as a transport vehicle for lipids that otherwise would not be soluble in blood or lymph.

High Density Lipoproteins (HDL)—Protein molecules that contain a lower amount of lipid as cholesterol. HDL returns lipids from the storage places to the liver for dismantling and disposal.

Low Density Lipoproteins (LDL)—Protein molecules that contain most of the cholesterol. They transport lipids from liver to other tissues such as muscle, mammary glands, etc.

Lymph—A pale coagulable fluid that bathes the tissues and consists of varying numbers of white blood cells and a few red blood cells.

Myocardium—The thick muscular layer of the heart wall.

Metabolism—All the chemical changes that occur from the time nutrients are absorbed until they are built into body substances or are excreted.

Nutrient—A substance obtained from food and used in the body to promote growth, maintenance, or repair.

Obesity—Body weight more than 15% to 25% above desirable weight; excessive body fatness.

Occlusion—Shutting off the blood flow in an artery.

Ophthalmia—Inflammation of the deeper structures of the eye.

Organic—A compound which contains carbon. (Unfortunately, this term is used very indiscriminately by some commercial retailers for sales purposes.)

Osteoarthritis—Degenerative disease characterized by the formation of calcium in the joints.

Osteoporosis—A disease of older persons in which the bones become porous and brittle.

Overweight—Body weight more than 10% above desirable weight.

Oxidation—The combining of a substance with oxygen.

Pancreas—A gland behind the stomach and between the spleen and small intestine. It secretes a number of digestive juices, as well as the hormone insulin which controls carbohydrate metabolism.

Pellagra—A niacin-deficiency disease.

Peristalsis—Progressive worm-like movement of food in the intestinal tract.

Plaque—A patch or small differentiated area on a body surface. In blood vessels, plaques are formed from deposits of cholesterol, fats, and calcium, fibrin, and platelet aggregation.

Platelet—A small disk-shaped structure in blood which is active in blood coagulation.

Pneumonia—Inflammation of the lungs.

Polychlorinated Biphenyls (PCB's)—Chlorinated organic industrial compounds that are toxic. They're gradually being phased out by industry, as they're freely dumped into rivers, contaminating drinking water.

Polyunsaturated Fat—A fat or oil which is generally from a plant source and liquid at room temperature.

Quadriceps—The four muscles in the front part of the thigh.

Radial Artery—An artery located in the forearm.

Refined—Refers to the process by which the coarse parts of certain food products are removed. For example, the refining of wheat into flour involves removing three of the four parts of the kernel—the chaff, the bran, and the germ, leaving only the endosperm (starch).

Rheumatic Heart Disease—A heart condition that occurs as a result of rheumatic fever. Rheumatic fever is caused by a streptococcus bacteria which may damage the heart valves so that blood cannot flow through them normally. Ranks among the leading causes of heart disease among children.

Roughage—Indigestible fibers of foods.

Saturated Fat—A fat which is generally from an animal source and solid at room temperature.

Shin Splints—Inflammation of the anterior tibial muscles, i.e., those muscles located in the shin area.

Sodium—Salt.

Stroke—Brain impairment due to hemorrhage in the brain or lesion in a blood vessel supplying the brain.

Sucrose—A disaccharide composed of glucose and fructose, commonly known as table sugar, beet sugar, or cane sugar.

Sugar—A monosaccharide or a disaccharide.

Synthesis—Process by which a new substance is formed from its individual parts.

Systolic (See Blood Pressure).

Tachycarida—Rapid beating of the heart, usually applied to rates over 100 per minute.

Tendon—Connective tissue attaching muscle to bone.

Thiamin—Vitamin B_1. Necessary for the normal flow of glucose from food to energy. Deficiency causes beriberi.

Thickening Agents—Natural or chemically modified carbohydrates that absorb some of the water that is present in food, thereby making the food thicker. Thickening agents "stabilize" factory-made foods by keeping the complex mixtures of oils, water, acids, and solids well mixed.

Thrombus—A clot in a blood vessel or in one of the cavities of the heart.

Triceps—The three muscles in the upper part of the back of the arm.

Trichinosis—Disease resulting from the ingestion of raw or inadequately cooked meat (especially pork) that contains small worms whose larvae infest the intestines and voluntary muscles of man. Symptoms consist of fever, nausea, diarrhea, and muscular pains.

Triglycerides—A type of fat containing three fatty acids; a major dietary lipid, as well as the body's storage form for food energy eaten in excess of need.

Trihalomethanes (THM's)—Three cancer-causing compounds that are formed in water when halogens (chlorine, bromine, and iodine) are added to water. Current Environmental Protective Agency (E.P.A.) limit is 100 parts per billion.

Urea—A product of protein metabolism, found in urine, blood, and lymph, that is eliminated from the body in the urine.

Uric Acid—A product of protein metabolism, insoluble in water, but soluble in alkaline solutions. Excessive amounts in the blood are associated with gout.

Vasodilation—Enlargement of the blood vessels.

Ventrical—Any of various cavities or hallow organs; specifically, a) either of the two lower chambers of the heart which receive blood from the auricles and pump it into the arteries; b) any of the four small continuous cavities within the brain.

Varicose Veins—Abnormal distention of veins most commonly seen in the legs, probably as a result of incomplete valves. There is a predisposition to varicose veins among persons in occupations requiring long periods of standing, and in pregnant women.

Vitamin—A potent, indispensable, noncaloric organic compound needed in small amounts in the diet, which performs specific and individual functions to promote growth or reproduction or to maintain health and life.

Index